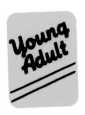

Opium

DRUGS The Straight Facts

■ DRUGS
The Straight Facts

Opium

Thomas M. Santella

Consulting Editor
David J. Triggle
University Professor
School of Pharmacy and Pharmaceutical Sciences
State University of New York at Buffalo

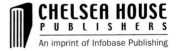

CHELSEA HOUSE
PUBLISHERS
An imprint of Infobase Publishing

Opium

Chelsea House
An imprint of Infobase Publishing
132 West 31st Street
New York NY 10001

Library of Congress Cataloging-in-Publication Data

Santella, Thomas M.
   Opium / Thomas M. Santella.
         p. cm — (Drugs: the straight facts)
   Includes bibliographical references and index.
   ISBN 0-7910-8547-3 (hardcover)
  1. Opium—Juvenile literature. I. Title. II. Series
   RM 666.O6S26 2006
   615'.32335—dc22   2006020612

Chelsea House books are available at special discounts when purchased in bulk quantities for businesses, associations, institutions, or sales promotions. Please call our Special Sales Department in New York at (212) 967-8800 or (800) 322-8755.

You can find Chelsea House on the World Wide Web at http://www.chelseahouse.com

Text and cover design by Terry Mallon, Keith Trego

Printed in the United States of America

Bang EJB 10 9 8 7 6 5 4 3 2 1

This book is printed on acid-free paper.

All links and web addresses were checked and verified to be correct at the time of publication. Because of the dynamic nature of the web, some addresses and links may have changed since publication and may no longer be valid.

Table of Contents

The Use and Abuse of Drugs

The issues associated with drug use and abuse in contemporary society are vexing subjects, fraught with political agendas and ideals that often obscure essential information that teens need to know to have intelligent discussions about how to best deal with the problems associated with drug use and abuse. *Drugs: The Straight Facts* aims to provide this essential information through straightforward explanations of how an individual drug or group of drugs works in both therapeutic and nontherapeutic conditions; with historical information about the use and abuse of specific drugs with discussion of drug policies in the United States; and with an ample list of further reading.

From the start, the series uses the word "drug" to describe psychoactive substance that are used for medicinal or non-medicinal purposes. Included in this broad category are substances that are legal or illegal. It is worth noting that humans have used many of these substances for hundreds, if not thousands of years. For example, traces of marijuana and cocaine have been found in Egyptian mummies; the use of peyote and Amanita fungi has long been a component of religious ceremonies worldwide; and alcohol production and consumption have been an integral part of many human culture's social and religious ceremonies. One can speculate about why early human societies chose to use such drugs. Perhaps, anything that could provide relief from the harshness of life—anything that could make the poor conditions and fatigue associated with hard work easier to bear—was considered a welcome tonic. Life was likely to be, according to seventeenth century English philosopher Thomas Hobbes, "poor, nasty, brutish, and short." One can also speculate about modern human societies' continued use and abuse of drugs. Whatever the reasons, the consequences of sustained drug use are not insignificant—addiction, overdose, incarceration, and drug wars—and must be dealt with by an informed citizenry.

The problem that faces our society today is how to break the connection between our demand for drugs and the willingness of largely outside countries to supply this highly profitable trade. This is the same problem we have faced since narcotics and cocaine were outlawed by the Harrison Narcotic Act of 1914, and we have yet to defeat it despite current expenditures of approximately $20 billion per year on "the war on drugs." The first step in meeting any challenge is always an intelligent and informed citizenry. The purpose of this series is to educate our readers so that they can make informed decisions about issues related to drugs and drug abuse.

SUGGESTED ADDITIONAL READING

Courtwright, David T. *Forces of Habit, Drugs and the Making of the Modern World.* Cambridge, Mass: Harvard University Press, 2001. David T. Courtwright is Professor of History at the University of North Florida.

Davenport-Hines, Richard. *The Pursuit of Oblivion, A Global History of Narcotics.* New York: Norton, 2002. The author is a professional historian and a member of the Royal Historical Society.

Huxley, Aldous. *Brave New World.* New York: Harper & Rowe, 1932. Huxley's book, written in 1932, paints a picture of a cloned society devoted only to the pursuit of happiness.

David J. Triggle, Ph.D.
University Professor
School of Pharmacy and Pharaceutical Sciences
State University of New York at Buffalo

1

A Brief History of Opium

Over the course of human history there have been countless powerful natural and artificial drugs, but none parallel **opium** in its mythical status, range of uses, and longevity of interest. Indeed, no other drug has had an economic, political, and social influence comparable to opium and its derivatives. Opium is the oldest drug ever cultivated and actively pursued by the human species; it even predates the fermentation of alcohol. The story of opium could fill entire libraries with historical, clinical, and anecdotal information.

The story of opium is one of both individual and global conflict. It is a story of alleviating pain and inspiring genius, of addiction, escape, and freedom, of contradictions and mystery. Above all, the story of opium is one of constant mutation within the instability and evolution of human consumption and addiction. The story is as relevant today as it was during the great opium wars of the mid-nineteenth century, yet it stretches back into the far reaches of human civilization.

EARLY OPIUM USE

The details of the earliest cultivation and use of opium for its euphoric effects are highly disputed, as it certainly predates the existence of written languages. Therefore, there are no physical records that date back to the beginnings of opium's use. Another difficulty in pinpointing the earliest use of opium is that it comes from the pod of a specific type of poppy plant called *Papaver somniferum*. In addition to being utilized for its narcotic aspects, the poppy has also traditionally been used (and is still used today) for its poppy seeds, which garnish breads and spice up salad dressings.

Despite these difficulties, experts generally agree that by 3400 B.C., opium was being cultivated around the Tigres-Euphrates river system, in lower Mesopotamia (what is now Iraq), by the Sumerian civilization. The Sumerians, who were responsible, among other things, for the creation of written language, called the plant Hul Gil, or "joy plant." While little is known about the extent to which the Sumerians used the plant as a drug, its designation as the "joy plant" suggests that its euphoric properties were recognized.

Just as the earliest cultivation of opium is disputed, so is the rate and method that spread opium use around the globe. It has long been assumed that knowledge of opium originated in Egypt, moved to Asia, and then made its way to the rest of Europe. However, archeological discoveries have led researchers to believe that, from Mesopotamia, opium use spread south and west, eventually making its way to Europe. According to this theory, opium would have been introduced to Asia much later than was earlier assumed. Regardless of its precise mode of diffusion, knowledge of opium was originally passed down from the Sumerians to the Assyrians, from the Assyrians to the Babylonians, and from the Babylonians to the Egyptians.

EGYPT

According to historical records, around 1500 B.C. the use of opium, as well as its exportation, was beginning to take root. The city of Thebes was so well-known for its poppy fields that it lent its name to the active alkaloid in opium, thebaine. **Alkaloids** are any of a host of organic compounds, often complex in structure, derived from plants. Many [alkaloids] are useful as medicines and poisons. In medical texts left by the Egyptians, there are more than 700 medicines that contain opium. Under the rule of Thutmose IV, Akhenaton, and Tutankhamen, the Egyptian opium trade expanded. Opium was sold by the Phoenicians and Minoans, and transported across the Mediterranean to Carthage, Greece, and the rest of Europe.

GREECE

In ancient Greece, the use of opium was well known, though principally for its mystical qualities. Priests were aware of the euphoric qualities of opium and imbued the drug with supernatural qualities. It was used in religious ceremonies and disseminated by priests to treat illness, and the healing effects of opium were formally recognized by Hippocrates (460–357 B.C.). Hippocrates is known as the "Father of Medicine." He advocated a less superstitious view of opium and was strongly in favor of a more scientific approach to its study. Hippocrates valued the medicinal qualities of opium over the religious uses, and viewed it as a useful medical tool for a host of conditions, particularly diarrhea.

As opium came to be recognized in Greek society for its medicinal and mystical qualities, it began to appear in the great literary works of the time. In Homer's *Odyssey*, it appeared under the name "nepenthe" as a drug of forgetfulness. Homer also described its use after a battle for soldiers mourning the loss of warriors killed in action. In these descriptions, Homer was drawing on experiences that were true to life and would have been recognized by fellow Greeks. As Greece continually fought for imperial power, its armies continued to spread knowledge of the mystical poppy.

ROME

The Romans also imbued opium with mythical meanings. Roman mythology was full of references to the effects of opium. Somnus, the Roman god of sleep, was often envisaged as a boy carrying a handful of opium plants. Ceres, the goddess of fertility, used the drug as a pain reliever. Perhaps the best evidence of

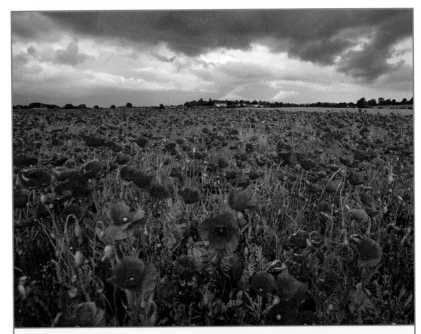

Figure 1.1 Poppy field. © Richard Cummins/CORBIS.

the influence of opium on Roman society can be seen on ancient currency. Roman coinage was emblazoned with a poppy, and used throughout the Roman empire. For the Romans, opium was both a medicinal and a recreational drug. For recreational purposes, the Romans ate the entire poppy pod, crushed and mixed with honey. Until relatively recent times, eating or drinking opium (pure or mixed with innumerable additives) was the principal form of its consumption.

OPIUM USE SPREADS

Though the Roman Empire was declining, the trade in opium was rapidly expanding. This spread was due in part to military exploits abroad, in addition to the influences of Arab scholars and medicine men, who were part of the most advanced societies of the time. By 330 B.C., Alexander the Great had advanced with his army into Persia and India, further opening up the channels of opium trade. After the death of Muhammad, in 632 A.D., the Arab Empire rapidly expanded its influence as far north as Spain, into east and west Africa, across Persia and India, and all the way to China. Following this movement of warriors, traders, and religious men was the indelible influence of opium. Arab societies held the reins of opium production and transport for the next eight or nine centuries, until Europeans would eventually transform the plant into a global commodity and a tool for economic exploitation.

OPIUM USE IN THE MODERN ERA

While the cultivation of opium continued to spread throughout the centuries, it experienced a notable transformation in the sixteenth century, as it increasingly became an international and domestic commodity of vast economic importance. The first country to exploit this advancing commodity was Portugal. In 1498, the Portuguese explorer Vasco da Gama made his way around the southernmost tip of Africa (the Cape of Good Hope), eventually reaching the city of Calcutta in India. As a result of this establishment of a secure trade route, Portugal was able to maintain a trade monopoly with India until 1600. One of the major items of trade was opium. Opium

WHAT'S IN A NAME? THE MEANING OF OPIUM

The word *opium* comes from the Greek *opos* (juice) or *opion* (poppy juice). According to the *Oxford English Dictionary*, opium is "a reddish-brown, strongly scented addictive drug prepared from the thickened dried latex of the unripe capsules of the opium poppy, *Papaver somniferum*, used illicitly as a narcotic, and occasionally medicinally as a sedative and analgesic."

was an ideal trading commodity because of its light weight, high price, and equally high demand.

Over the next 100 years, a struggle ensued between various European powers, including the Dutch, French, and British, over control of the opium trade. By 1715, it was clear that Britain had won when it secured the port of Canton, the only port through which opium could be sold to China. The disheartening and complex relationship between Britain and China involving opium will be explored in much greater detail later.

For the countries of Europe, opium was a critical product for trade with the countries of the Far East. The problem for the Europeans (a problem Americans eventually encountered as well) was that while they increasingly required goods from the Far East, such as tea and especially silk, countries like China were not equally interested in Western goods. But the Chinese *were* interested in opium, an interest that provided Europe with the leverage for effective trade. For Europeans, especially the British, this meant that they had to control the trade in places where opium could be grown, such as India. This need for control lead to the creation of Britain's infamous East India Company.

The need for opium was not unique to China. Indeed, opium was more than a primary product of international trade; it became an essential commodity in Europe as well.

OPIUM IN BRITAIN AND AMERICA

By 1830, Britain's dependence on opium was at its highest levels ever, with consumption reaching 22,000 pounds of opium in that year. The ethos of opium use in Britain over the course of the nineteenth century is illuminated in the writings of countless prominent literary figures. In 1819, poet John Keats was openly experimenting with opium as a recreational "muse" for his writings. In 1822, Thomas De Quincey published his now infamous *Confessions of an English Opium-Eater*, the most revealing autobiographical account of opium addiction to date. The British poet Elizabeth Barrett Browning was experimenting with **morphine** (opium's active ingredient) by 1837.

At the same time that opium was increasing its hold on English society, scientists were advancing the potency and delivery of the drug, thereby enhancing its euphoric qualities. In 1803, German scientist Friedrich Sertürner isolated the active ingredient in opium, morphine. This discovery was lauded by physicians because it enhanced their ability to control the drug's effects for treating illness. By 1827, Germany's E. Merck & Company was manufacturing morphine commercially for medical use. In 1843, a new technique for morphine delivery was invented, whereby morphine was injected directly into the bloodstream with a syringe, tripling its potency. Finally, in 1874, British scientist C. R. Wright synthesized heroin (also known as diacetylmorphine) by boiling morphine with acetic acid. Wright could not have realized that heroin would become the twentieth century's most lethal and widespread narcotic.

In the nineteenth century, the potency and use of opium increased across Europe and Asia, and its lethal grasp began to take root in America. In 1840, 24,000 pounds of opium were exported to New England, resulting in the government's taxation of the product (opium was not yet illegal in America). By the late 1800s, opium use in America was overtaken by the more potent power of heroin. Originally used as a cure for morphine addiction, heroin posed an equal, if not substantially greater, potential for addiction.

As a result, the temperance movement in the United States. in the early twentieth century led to increased legislation to curb the use of opium and its derivatives. In 1905, the U.S. Congress banned the sale of opium, and the Harrison Narcotics Act of 1917 required patients to receive prescriptions for potentially harmful drugs. By 1923, most narcotic substances, including heroin and morphine, were banned from over-the-counter sale.

But these regulations were not successful in eliminating the abuse of opium and its derivatives. Global conflicts and changing trading venues resulted in ups and downs in the consumption of opium across the globe, but opium (primarily in the form of heroin) continues to be a major trade commodity with sales in the billions of dollars per year. Hundreds of thousands, perhaps millions, of addicts around the world continue to battle the unrelenting power of heroin to this day.

2

Opium: From Poppy Plant to Heroin

THE POPPY PLANT

The opium poppy, or **Papaver somniferum**, is just one of more than 100 different poppy plant species that grow both in the wild and in cultivated settings around the world. While *P. somniferum* is one of many different poppies, it is one of only two species that produce morphine (the active ingredient in opium) and the only one actively cultivated to produce the drug.

There is great debate as to why the opium poppy produces the alkaloids that it does (see "The Active Substances in Opium" box). What purpose does it serve? Some experts believe that these chemicals are created by the plant as a form of protection against animal predators. Others maintain that the alkaloids are essential in the production of the plants seeds. A third and very intriguing theory holds that the high concentration of morphine and other alkaloids in *P. somniferum* is a product of its reaction to human cultivation. In other words, as humans increasingly planted the opium poppy for its medicinal and narcotic qualities, they naturally targeted the plants with the highest concentrations of morphine. Successful cultivators were those with the most plants containing the highest levels of narcotic. Thus, over thousands of years of selecting the most potent plants, humans have evolved the opium poppy to their own needs. Still, the real reason for the plant's excessive alkaloid production remains a mystery. In fact, experts have yet to even identify the mechanism by which the plant produces the alkaloids.

THE ACTIVE SUBSTANCES IN OPIUM

Contrary to what its name suggests, opium is not a single chemical compound. Its chemical make-up is more like a salad, consisting of various substances including sugars, proteins, acids, water, and many alkaloids, among others. The people who grow opium for its narcotic value are primarily interested in the alkaloids.

An alkaloid is a complex organic chemical substance found in plants, which characteristically combines nitrogen with other elements, has a bitter taste, and typically has some toxic, stimulant, analgesic effects. There are many different alkaloids, 30 of which are found in the opium plant. While morphine is the most important alkaloid in opium—for its natural narcotic qualities as well as providing the chemical structure for heroin—another alkaloid, codeine, is also sought after for its medicinal attributes. Other alkaloids include papaverine, narcotine, nicotine, atropine, cocaine, and mescaline. While the concentration of morphine in opium varies depending on where and how the plant is cultivated, it typically ranges from 3 percent to 20 percent.

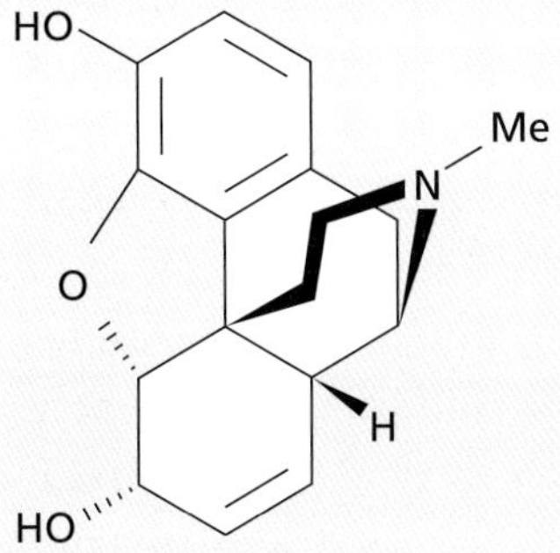

Morphine

© Infobase Publishing

Figure 2.1 Chemical structure of morphine.

From a horticultural standpoint, the opium **poppy** is quite a beautiful plant. The poppy is a tall, thin plant of about 90–150 centimeters with little surrounding its stem. When in bloom, its four sprouting leaves can be a variety of colors—white, pink, blue, crimson, or any combination of these. These leaves surround the plant's inner pod. The pod has three layers, including an outer wall and inner compartments where its seeds are produced. Typically about the size of a golf ball, the pod contains the plant's two major products: the seeds (about 1,000 for every plant), which can be cultivated into new plants, and opium.

THE GROWING PROCESS

Perhaps part of opium's success as a cultivated narcotic is the relative ease with which it can be grown. The opium poppy is an annual with a 120-day growth cycle. Opium can be grown under disparate soil conditions, but a dark rich soil that has been well farmed and is loose enough to allow the roots of the plant to set in is best. The poppy prefers a temperate climate with long days of sun and moderate rain. During the growth cycle, the plant needs relatively little attention and it does not require irrigation or expensive pesticides. The poppy is also capable of replanting on its own as wind blows the seeds to the ground. However, planters usually collect the seeds themselves and replant them in rows.

Once planted, the poppy plant grows rapidly. After six weeks, the roots are well established and the plant begins to sprout. By the eighth week, the plant may be as high as 60 centimeters with the pod firmly established. As the growth cycle progresses, insects carry out fertilization and the plant grows taller while developing its four colored petals and characteristic central pod, from which the resin for opium is extracted.

Opium cultivation is widespread but mostly centered in the subtropical regions of the northern hemisphere. Specifically, the most important opium-producing regions in the world are: Southeast Asia, which is believed to produce 70 percent of the

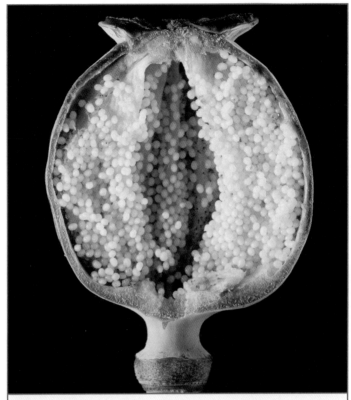

Figure 2.2 Poppy seeds inside pod. © Dr. Jeremy Burgess/Photo Researchers, Inc.

world's opium; West Asia, producing about 25 percent; South America, particularly Colombia, which produces 5 percent and finally Mexico with 1 percent.

Notably 85 percent of all opium cultivation is directed toward illicit commerce. Most opium is converted into heroin before it is put on the market. This is the result of several factors. First, to produce the same effect, it requires approximately 30 times more opium than heroin. Also, heroin takes up less space and is thus easier and safer to smuggle. Finally, heroin, because of its more powerful and concentrated effect, can be sold at greater prices, earning the dealer higher profits than with opium.

Table 2.1 The International Language of Poppy

Language	Poppy Name
Bengali	Afing-gach, Posto
Burmese	Bhainzi
Dutch	Papaver
English	Poppy
French	Pavot somnifere
German	Mohnblume
Hindi	Post, Khas-khas, Post dana
Hungarian	Mak, Kerti mak
Italian	Papavero
Japanese	Hinageshi
Polish	Mak lekarski
Portuguese	Popoula
Romanian	Mac
Sanskrit	Ahiphena
Spanish	Adormidera, Amapola
Swedish	Vallmo
Thai	Ton fin
Turkish	Hashhash tohuma

Adapted from Moraes, Francis, and Debra Moraes. *Opium*. Oakland, Calif.: Ronin Publishing, 2003.

EXTRACTING THE OPIUM

The extraction of opium from the poppy is an arduous and laborious task, which has changed very little for thousands of years. When fully grown, each plant must be attended to personally by the planter in a process referred to as tapping (also called scoring). The difficulty of this task is increased by the fact that not all of the plants will be ready to harvest at the same time, thus the planter must pay close attention and mark each plant as he or she goes.

When ready, the planter taps the pod with a small, three- or four-bladed knife, making vertical lacerations. The grower

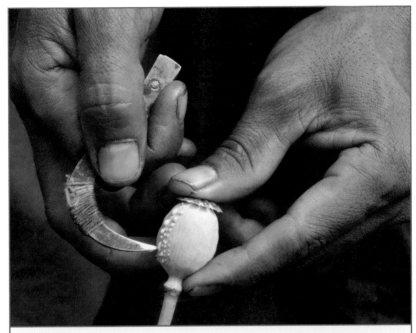

Figure 2.3 Person scoring poppy pod to get resin. © Michael Freeman/CORBIS

then waits for the opium resin to seep out of the pod. As this can take several hours, the grower usually taps the plants at dusk and then returns the following morning. The planter must be careful not to cut too deeply into the pod, as that would cause the plant to die. He cannot cut too shallow, either, or the plant will form a scab over the laceration, preventing any opium collection.

Once the resin has caramelized on the outer surface of the pod, the planter, using a small, blunt-edged tool, will scrape off the resin and collect it in a pail attached to his waist. This process will be done perhaps half a dozen times for each plant, with a total collection of around 80 milligrams of opium per plant. Opium cultivators working on legal farms that produce the raw materials for pharmaceuticals clean the scraping blade between each plant. However, most of the world's growers lick

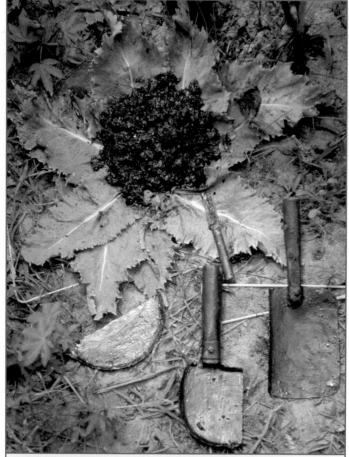

Figure 2.4 Raw opium and harvesting hand tools.
© Francoise de Mulder/CORBIS

the blade to clean it and literally become addicted to their crops.

PREPARATION FOR MARKET

Once the opium has been collected from the plant, it is far from ready to be sold to traders or turned into heroin. In its raw state, opium is brown and has a gummy paste-like consistency, and it must be dried for several days as it contains a great deal of water. After this initial drying period, the opium gum is flattened into cakes, rolled into balls, or molded into any number of shapes, depending on the personal preference of the farmer. The opium is then wrapped in plastic and stored for several months. Over time, the molded opium continues to dry and hardens, allowing it to become as concentrated as possible. But even after months of drying, the opium will still contain a certain amount of impurities, such as additional plant matter that was mixed in when the plant was initially

OPIUM GROWING FOR LEGAL MEDICINAL PURPOSES

While opium is illegal in most countries in the world, including the United States, there are many lawful farming operations. These farms produce the products used by the pharmaceutical industry to make a variety of medications. While only an estimated 15 percent of all opium poppy farming is directed toward legal ends, the chemical substances produced are very important and include

- Morphine
- Codeine
- Dihydrocodeine
- Hydrocodone
- Thebaine
- Oxycodone
- Ethylmorphine

These drug products are used in a number of ways to treat various medical conditions, including the common cough, diarrhea, and pain. Surgeons and dentists also use morphine, the most important chemical substance within the opium poppy, as an anesthetic. Unfortunately, most opium is turned into heroin and ends up in the veins of addicts.

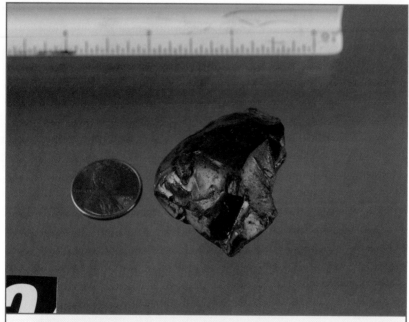

Figure 2.5 Raw opium. © Courtesy Drug Enforcement Administration

tapped. As a result of these impurities, the opium must be cooked before being sold.

The dried opium is dissolved in boiling water to remove remaining impurities, and any plant matter is left floating on the top. The liquid is then sifted through a fine cloth or sieve, thus removing any larger particles. What remains is pure liquid opium, which is left simmering until it becomes a thick, brown paste. Once again, the dried paste is molded and wrapped. After this long process, the highly concentrated opium is ready to be sold to traders, smoked by addicts, or turned into heroin or other pharmaceuticals like codeine.

Although the poppy plant's active ingredients are tapped and turned into opium for export, farmers typically do not waste the rest of the plant. The seeds, which develop in the pod even after it is tapped, contain no toxic substances and are edible

(Figure 2.2). These seeds are valuable and used to garnish a host of food products, including desserts, breads, and salad dressings. These seeds also yield an oil that can be used for cooking or as the base for oil paints. Perhaps the most important function of the seeds is to grow more poppy plants which fuel the never-ending cycle of opium production, a cycle that has existed for centuries and has led to enumerable conflicts throughout history.

3

The Economics of Opium: Trade, Consumption, and War

OPIUM TRADE BEGINS

By the sixteenth century, the market for opium was well established across Europe, Asia, and North Africa. For the first time, Persians and Indians began using opium as a recreational drug, vastly widening its market potential. As far back as the eighth century, Arab traders sold opium to China as a medicinal product and recreational drug. China, with a long history of opium use for its medicinal qualities and with its massive population, was the center of the global opium trade from the fifteenth through the nineteenth centuries.

It was the Portuguese who first realized and capitalized on the sale of opium, establishing a trade in the early sixteenth century. The Portuguese initially sold tobacco from their Brazilian colony in exchange for China's silk. Like other European nations, Portugal quickly discovered that opium provided a much better tool for trade. The problem for Portugal, as for the Dutch, British, and Americans who followed, was that China, with its large population and ample arable land, did not require any particular Western goods. The West, however, increasingly sought China's precious silk and tea, but

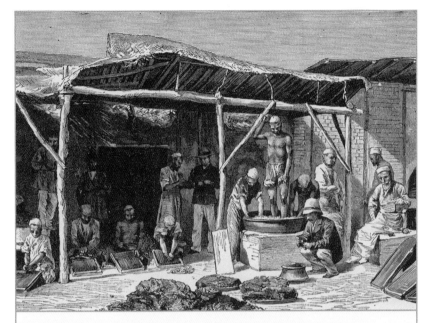

Figure 3.1 Indian opium manufactory. Hierophant Collection

needed an equivalent trading commodity. Opium, as a highly addictive product that could grow almost anywhere, proved a perfect product for exchange.

Dutch merchants were quick to enter the increasingly lucrative opium trade. The Dutch, like the Portuguese, focused their efforts on controlling the Chinese market. By securing monopolies in India through the Dutch East India Company, the trade expanded rapidly. By the late 1600s, the Dutch were buying massive quantities of cheap opium from India (87 tons in 1699) and turning profits of 400 percent through its sale in China. The opium trade grew extensively over the sixteenth and early seventeenth centuries, creating swaths of Chinese opium addicts and prompting the Chinese Emperor to ban opium for the first time in 1729. However, the opium trade was simply too lucrative to resist. Over the next century, the British transformed opium from a relatively limited luxury item into a global commodity.

FROM LUXURY TO COMMODITY

During the first centuries of the opium trade, the drug became popular not only in Asia but in the Western world as well. In Britain, especially, opium became an extremely important product, both within the country and for its economic attributes abroad. For much of this time, the British attitude toward opium was much like our modern view of coffee. The English, along with much of the rest of the Western world, viewed opium as a luxury and a pleasantry, albeit a mildly addictive one. Like coffee today, opium was realized to be mildly addictive, but it was not seen as a dangerous narcotic.

Opium was, in fact, widely used in British society. It was sold in pharmacies and prescribed by doctors as a remedy for all sorts of ills. Opium was combined with liquor and sold in bars. A bottle of this popular mixture of opium and liquor, called **laudanum**, was commonplace in English households (see "Sydenham's Laudanum" box). While the English opinion of opium eventually changed, its initial acceptance as a rather harmless luxury item might have given merchants a clear conscious when pushing its sale on China.

SYDENHAM'S LAUDANUM

Invented in 1527, laudanum, a designation for a number of products containing opium, liquor, and a variety of other ingredients, was the most popular form of opium consumption in the West. Of all the laudanum products available, the most popular was a brand called Sydenham's Laudanum, which contained one pound of sherry wine, two ounces of opium, one ounce of saffron, one ounce of powder of cinnamon, and one ounce of powder of cloves. Its popularity stemmed from the sweetness of the sherry undercutting the natural bitterness of opium. For more than 400 years, this method of opium drinking remained widespread among Western nations.

THE ROAD TO WAR

By 1773, the British East India Company (BEIC), which effectively made India a British colony, had taken over the opium trade with China from the Dutch. That year, the British Governor-General of Bengal eliminated all competing sources of opium production in India, making Bengal the capital of opium production. The Governor, with a monopoly on Indian opium, established the system by which the trade flourished for the next century. Interestingly, the Governor made it illegal for BEIC ships to carry opium for sale in China. This was done because the sale of opium to China was technically illegal. The Chinese government had banned opium smoking in 1729 and made its importation illegal in 1799.

Despite these laws, the British continued to smuggle opium through clandestine operations. Rather than directly loading British ships, which sailed to Chinese ports, the opium grown in Bengal was sold to private (British) merchants, who could then carry the opium on their personal vessels for sale at local Chinese auctions. In 1797, the BEIC ousted local opium buyers in Bengal, leaving the British government as the sole proprietor of Indian opium. By the end of the 18th century, Britain controlled the cultivation, processing, export, and sale of opium to China.

Despite the fact that selling opium to China was illegal, the British transformed the product from a relatively limited luxury good into a major commodity. Throughout the nineteenth century, the British continually expanded the growth capacity of the opium fields in Bengal. At its height, the opium fields consisted of 500,000 acres of prime land, employing over a million farmers who grew and sent massive quantities of opium to the British-controlled processing factories in Patna and Benares. At the factories, the opium was processed and made ready for export. Once molded into balls, the opium was packed into chests (140 pounds each), sealed, and sold to private British merchants.

With a seemingly unlimited addict population in China, the sale of opium became a major source of income for the British, constituting much of their tax revenue from India and completely paying for Chinese tea sent to Britain. For many years, the BEIC set the amount of opium sold to China at 4,000 chests (280 tons). During this time, the British did not desire or make a profit but simply sold enough opium to take care of their need for China's tea. However, the demand for opium in China far outstretched the artificially set British supply, causing competition from Turkey, west India, and America.

When the BEIC lost its monopoly on Indian opium in 1834, the trade grew exponentially, with each nation clawing for control over China's growing market. The intense competition led to the development of a new fleet of ships, called "**opium clippers**," which could carry more opium and travel faster, to undercut the competition (see "The Opium Clipper" box). All of this resulted in an expanding drug problem in China. By the 1830s, with a host of nations vying for control over the trade and producing and selling as much opium as possible, and with more than 3 million opium addicts in China, the Chinese government began to take more aggressive actions against the trade.

THE OPIUM CLIPPER

In the mid-1800s, with opium now a prized commodity, fierce competition and a growing Chinese market meant that speed of delivery increasingly determined profit. As a result, a new kind of ship was developed specifically for the transport and sale of opium. The "opium clippers" were designed to hold large amounts of cargo while sailing quickly enough to reduce costs and outrun pirates and competitors.

THE OPIUM WARS

By the 1830s, the Chinese government was becoming increasingly adamant about stopping the British opium trade. At the time, with more than 2,500 tons of opium imported each year, and with millions of addicts, opium had developed into a national epidemic. At first, the Emperor (Kea King) attempted to curb opium use by increasing the punishment for smoking from bamboo lashes to imprisonment and even death. But the trade continued undisturbed, in part because Chinese customs officials were consistently bribed and continued to allow the drug into the country. In 1836, the Emperor stepped up his anti-opium efforts by issuing an edict naming nine of the primary opium dealers and calling for their removal from the country. That effort also proved ineffective.

With relations becoming more embittered between the two governments, the Emperor tried to convince the Queen of England to stop the dreadful trade. In a letter sent to Queen Victoria, the Emperor pleaded to the Queen's sense of decency, writing: "If you will persist in selling your opium . . . there is not a good or upright man whose head and heart will not burn with indignation at your conduct." Whether the Queen read and dismissed the letter (or whether it even made it to her), is unknown, but the sale of opium continued, further escalating the situation.

The Emperor, now more determined than ever, sent a Commissioner Lin to Canton (the principal opium port) with the authority to stop the trade. Lin made the Emperor's wishes known, first by executing a Chinese opium smuggler. Lin then proceeded in blocking the port and forcing the traders to hand over their opium supplies, which were summarily destroyed. In blocking the port, Lin had also trapped around 300 British traders inside the city, and he threatened them with execution if they did not turn over their opium. Ultimately, tensions between the two nations rose to a fever pitch, and war was declared in November of 1839.

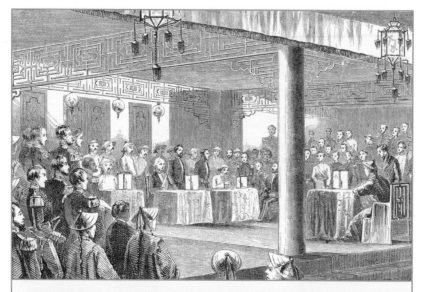

Figure 3.2 Signing of the Treaty of Tientsin. © Bettmann/CORBIS

The first opium war ended quickly, and in 1842 the defeated Chinese signed the Treaty of Nanking. According to the treaty's provisions, the British agreed to dissuade smugglers from selling opium. The treaty also forced the Chinese to open up five additional ports to the British, and required China to pay 4.5 million pounds to Britain for the destruction of its opium and the cost of the war. In addition, Britain gained the island of Hong Kong, which was subsequently used to stockpile opium on its way to market on the mainland. With the opium trade firmly reestablished, tensions mounted once again, leading to a second conflict in 1857.

The second opium war was characterized by increased British forces, resulting in a more violent conflict. Some reports estimated that in one battle, involving the British storming the port of Canton, 10,000 Chinese had been captured or killed within 10 minutes. Further reports indicated that within one 27-hour period, large swaths of Canton were torched, and the homes of nearly 30,000 people were burned. However, even after a decisive British victory at Canton, the Chinese refused to negotiate a new treaty. This defiance pushed the British to move their army toward the Chinese capital of Peking.

The Chinese, in order to avoid a repeat of Canton in the capital, agreed to sign a new treaty, the Treaty of Tientsin, on June 26, 1858. The new treaty, once ratified, legalized the sale and use of opium in China once and for all. Thus, by 1858, the opium trade was in full swing. As a global commodity, the drug became a critical component to the economies of exporting nations like Britain, which depended on the consistent revenue garnered through its high demand. The consumers were dependent on opium too, as the addictive properties proved too much for the masses of addicts to withstand.

4

The Chemical and Addictive Properties of Opium

Although the pharmacological and therapeutic properties of morphine represent the most widely studied aspects of the effects of opium, it must be recognized that opium is not a single chemical entity. Rather, it is a complex mixture of alkaloids with varying chemical and biological properties. It is the total sum of these biological effects that constitute the overall effects of opium. Although chemically diverse, all opium alkaloids share the ability to target specifically and impact the nervous system in both its peripheral and central components. An elementary understanding of the nervous system is therefore critical to an understanding of the effects of opium, as well as its alkaloid contents and synthetic analogs of morphine.

OPIUM AND THE NERVOUS SYSTEM

Although the nervous system is often discussed in terms of peripheral and central components, it should be regarded as a highly integrated whole in which the central nervous system (brain and spinal cord) plays a critical information gathering and processing role. The peripheral nervous system is often divided into the autonomic and somatic components. The somatic system controls the voluntary functions of the body, like those of the skeletal muscles. The

Table 4.1 The Principal Alkaloids in Opium

Alkaloid	Chemical Class	Amount in Opium
Morphine	Phenanthrene	10%–15%
Noscapine	Benzylisoquinoline	4%–8%
Codeine	Phenanthrene	1%–3%
Papaverine	Benzylisoquinoline	1%–3%
Thebaine	Phenanthrene	1%–2%

Adapted from Moraes, Francis, and Debra Moraes. *Opium*. Oakland, Calif.: Ronin Publishing, 2003, p. 58.

autonomic system, in contrast, is often referred to as the "involuntary" system. It regulates parts of the body where we execute little or no conscious control, such as the heart, intestines, vasculature, and other internal organs.

The autonomic nervous system is divided into the sympathetic and parasympathetic components, which typically exert opposing effects. The sympathetic system is involved in the "fight or flight" reaction (increased blood pressure and heart rate, and accommodation for increased vision, for example) that prepares the organism for stressful situations. The parasympathetic system conversely establishes a more relaxed situation, for instance, the rest period after a meal. The autonomic nervous system that is responsible for the independent control of the mechanical and secretory functions of the gastrointestinal tract is sometimes called the enteric system.

Drugs that affect the central nervous system may also have a major action in the gut. Thus, the constipating effects of opium alkaloids are exerted through this system and a number of the important withdrawal symptoms reflect the actions of the enteric nervous system. The nervous system is often regarded as a command (efferent) system that sends instructions to be executed. However, there is also a sensory (afferent) component, that receives information from innervated systems

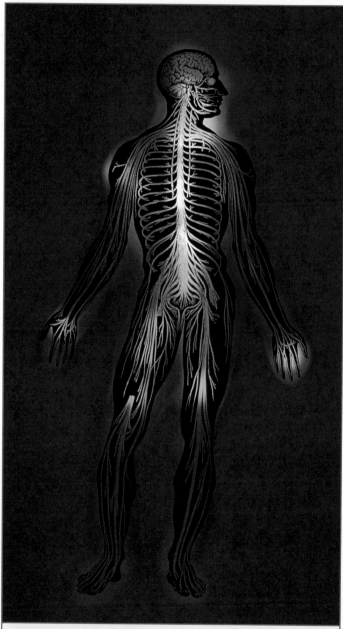

Figure 4.1 The nervous system. © M. Kulyk/Photo Researchers, Inc.

and that is vital to the overall integrated nervous response. Despite the anatomical and functional differences between the various components of the nervous system, they share a fundamental similarity in their use of chemicals (neurotransmitters) to convey information.

The individual unit of the nervous system is the neuron, a specialized cell that both receives and transmits information. The nervous system contains more than 100 billion neurons and is a major user of metabolic energy in the human body. It is also a region particularly susceptible to injury from toxic chemicals, lack of oxygen, and other assaults. Depending on the nervous region in which they reside, neurons may have different anatomical features and may use different chemical transmitters. Neurons communicate with each other and with their end organs by these chemical signals, which are released from the nerve terminal and interact with specific receptors on adjacent neurons or cells.

The chemical transmitters may be small molecules—notably acetylcholine, norepinephrine, epinephrine, serotonin, dopamine, or histamine. Acetylcholine and norpeinephrine are the dominant neurotransmitters in the parasympathetic and sympathetic nervous systems, respectively. Dopamine and serotonin are employed primarily in the central nervous system. Neurotransmitters may also be more complex peptides (small proteins) such as substance P, vasopressin, endorphins, and enkephalins. The latter agents are of particular importance to our considerations of opium since they represent the "endogenous" opiates—agents that exist within the body whose actions are mimicked by exogenous, or outside, agents such as morphine, heroin, codeine, and so on. These neurotransmitters serve to convey information between neurons across the synaptic cleft (the junction where two neurons meet) or at the neuroeffector junction (the site between neuron and an innervated organ such as muscle or secretory gland).

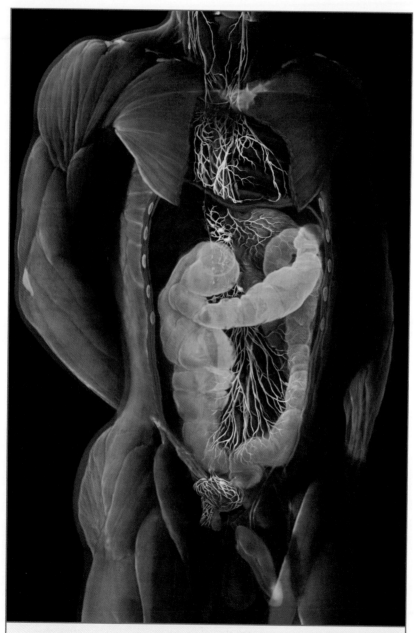

Figure 4.2 The autonomic nervous system. © Anatomical Travelogue/Photo Researchers, Inc.

Each neuron has specific synthetic machinery that enables it to both synthesize and eliminate a specific neurotransmitter. For example, neurons of the sympathetic nervous system employ norepinephrine and epinephrine as their transmitters. Other neurons, particularly in the central nervous system, employ dopamine as their transmitter. Dopamine is a particularly important transmitter for a variety of neuronal functions. Its loss is associated with Parkinson disease, and it is a critical agent in the mediation of pleasure and reward processes. Dopamine, due to its association with pleasurable sensations, is widely implicated in the actions of a number of drugs of abuse, including cocaine, opiates, and methamphetamines.

PHARMACOLOGICAL AND OPIOID RECEPTORS

It has been recognized for more than a century that the neurotransmitters of the nervous system produce their biological effects through interaction at specific drug binding sites or receptors. These receptors, many of which have been isolated and characterized in the past two decades, are typically specialized proteins on the cell surface. The function of these proteins is to recognize the neurotransmitter and to enable the molecule to bind to the receptor to trigger a biological response—muscle contraction, hormone or neurotransmitter secretion, or increased cardiac rate, for example. These interactions are typically quite specific and are often viewed in terms of a "lock and key" model. Despite this specificity it is usually found that a number of chemical variations around a particular structure can also be accommodated at the receptor site. When these chemical variants can also trigger the biological response they are termed "agonists." However, some molecules can bind to the receptor and not trigger the response, but rather block the response: these drugs are termed "antagonists." Thus, for example, the naturally occurring atropine from the Belladonna plant can block the actions of the neurotransmitter acetylcholine in

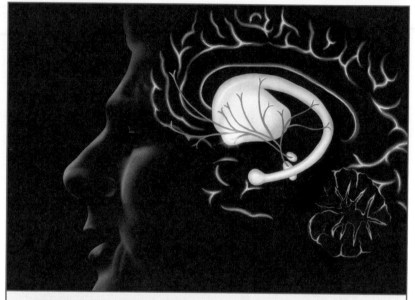

Figure 4.3 Dopamine release in the brain. © Bryson/Custom Medical Stock Photo

the parasympathetic system by interacting with the same receptors that acetylcholine uses.

The alkaloids in opium, including morphine, also interact with specific receptors (opiate receptors) within the central and peripheral nervous systems. At these receptors, the alkaloids in opium mimic the effects of the body's natural opiates. There are actually three major structural classes of opiates that occur in the body: enkephalins, endorphins, and dynorphins. The existence of these endogenous molecules was initially theorized because morphine and related drugs had been shown to exert their pharmacological and therapeutic effects through interaction at specific receptors. Due to the specific locations of these interactions, scientists postulated that there must exist corresponding endogenous physiologically employed molecules. A similar argument was employed in the search for the endogenous equivalent of the cannabinoids found in

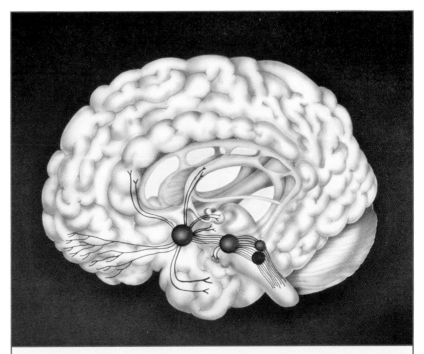

Figure 4.4 Brain showing binding sites and pathways of opiate drugs. © Kairos, Latin Stock/Photo Researchers, Inc.

marijuana and led to the recognition of the so-called "endo-cannabinoid" system.

There are three principal classes of opiate receptors, designated μ, κ, and δ, and there exist a number of drugs that are specific for each of these receptor types. However, most of the clinically used opiates are quite selective for the μ receptor: the endogenous opiates enkephalin, endorphin and dynorphin are selective for the μ and δ, δ and κ receptors respectively. When activated by opioids these receptors produce biochemical signals that block neurotransmitter release from nerve terminals, a process that underlies their blockade of pain signaling pathways as well as other effects, such as constipation, diuresis, euphoria, and feeding.

Brief administration of opioids leads to the development of acute tolerance, whereby increased quantities of the opioid are required to produce the same end result, but this process is rapidly reversed once the administration is ceased. However, more prolonged administration leads to classical or chronic tolerance from which state recovery to full sensitivity make take several days. These phenomena are not unique to opioid drugs, but rather are common to virtually all drug-receptor interactions and appear to be a common property of pharmacological receptors. Tolerance may also be associated with the state of physical dependence. The chronic administration of a drug, in this context an opioid, may result in a resetting of homeostatic mechanisms, and maintenance of this new state requires continued drug administration. Cessation of drug administration can then result in the phenomenon of withdrawal, during which the nervous system is excessively perturbed as it readapts to its original drug-free state. It should be emphasized that tolerance and physical dependence are physiological responses to continued administration of opioids and are not, contrary to some popular opinion, predictors of addiction. For example, patients with severe pain from bone cancer require very large amounts of opioids, yet these patients do not become addicted and will not even show withdrawal if the drug doses are reduced slowly over a period of days. Unfortunately, misinformation about opioids has led to patients with severe pain being undertreated.

ACTIVE INGREDIENTS IN OPIUM

Seventy-five percent of raw opium consists of ingredients that have no significant biological effects, such as water, sugars, and fatty acids. The remaining 25 percent contains numerous biologically active ingredients that interact with opioid receptors. These agents are termed the opiod alkaloids. Alkaloids are complex organic molecules, many of which have been used in traditional medicine or as poisons. Atropine from the deadly nightshade plant dilates the pupil of the eye, and curare is a skeletal muscle relaxant employed in anesthesia, but both agents have also been used as poisons. Opium contains at least 20 alkaloids and by some claims as many as 50. However, five principal alkaloids are of major interest: these are morphine, codeine, noscapine, papaverine, and thebaine.

Morphine is the most abundant of the opium alkaloids. It constitutes as much as 15 percent of the plant extract. Morphine has been used as a medicine and narcotic for thousands of years. Therapeutically, morphine has three principal uses: as an analgesic for the relief of acute and chronic pain, as a respiratory depressant, and as an antidiarrheal agent. The analgesic properties are morphine's most important clinical use.

Codeine is a close chemical relative of morphine, differing in only one chemical group. Once administered, codeine is actually metabolized by enzymatic action, and its actions mimic those of morphine. Codeine is used primarily as a cough suppressant, although it certainly also possesses significant analgesic properties (approximately one tenth those of morphine) as in the relief of pain from toothache.

Noscapaine has only minimal therapeutic and narcotic properties. It can be used as a cough suppressant, but has no apparent advantage over other agents.

Papaverine also has minimal narcotic properties. However, it does have vasodilator (blood vessel relaxant) properties, and because of this property it has been employed for both cognition enhancement and erectile dysfunction.

Thebaine has, despite its chemical similarity to morphine, no narcotic or therapeutic uses. It does, however, cause convulsions at high doses. It is also a useful chemical intermediate in the laboratory for production of other opioid compounds.

Table 4.2 Other Constituents of Opium

Constituent	Effects
Alpha-allocryptopine	Anti-arrhythmia, local anesthetic, antibacterial
Berberine	Fever reducer, inhibits protein formation
Canadine	Antibacterial, sedative
Coptisine	Antibacterial, antiinflammatory
Corytuberine	Causes seizures
Cryptopine	Anti-arrhythmia
Dihydrosanguinarine	Increases blood pressure
Isoboline	Antimicrobial
Isocorypalmine	Limits blood platelets
Laudanine	Increases respiration
Laudanosine	Principle metabolite in atracurium
Magnofluorine	Anti-inflammatory
Narceine	Similar to codeine
Narcotoline	Cough suppressant
Neopine	Like codeine, highly toxic
Oripavine	Analgesic, highly toxic
Protopine	Anti-arrhythmia
Pseudomorphine	No effect
Reticuline	Dopamine inhibitor
Rhoeadine	Mild sedative
Saguinarine	Raises blood pressure, antimicrobial, slows tumor growth, combats tooth decay
Salutaridine	Stimulates GABA receptors
Scoulerine	Sedative
Stepholidine	Analgesic, lowers blood pressure

5

"God's Own Medicine" or Drowsy Demon?

While opium invites a rather pallid perception today, it has historically been characterized as a wonderful writer's muse and incredibly useful medicine, as well as a terrible and evil drug that consumes and destroys its victims. Writing in the seventeenth century, the famous English physician Thomas Sydenham said of opium, "Among the remedies which it has pleased Almighty God to give to man to relieve his sufferings, none is so universal and so efficacious as opium." In the now infamous *Confessions of an English Opium Eater*, author Thomas De Quincey reflected, "Thou hast the keys of paradise, O just, subtle, and all-conquering opium." (See "Thomas De Quincey" box.) Indeed, countless writers have elevated opium to almost mythical status. Writing in the nineteenth century, influential Canadian physician and teacher Sir William Osler famously called opium "God's own medicine."

But others have deplored opium as nothing short of a drowsy demon. Writing about China in the late 1800s, John Thomson noted, "Smokers while asleep are like corpses, lean and haggard as demons. Opium-smoking throws whole families into ruin, dissipates every kind of property, and ruins man himself." Although countless writers have glorified opium smoking, exploring its reality uncovers a different, and perhaps less endearing, tale.

THOMAS DE QUINCEY

Born in 1785 in Manchester, England, Thomas De Quincey is recognized as a great English author, essayist, critic, and philosopher. Of all of his writings though, his most famous (and infamous) was *Confessions of an English Opium Eater*, published in 1821. In a bold move for his time, *Confessions* is an autobiographical account of De Quincey's use of opium to treat depression, his subsequent addiction, his artistic rivalry with the poet Samuel Taylor Coleridge, and his painstaking efforts to loosen the drug's grasp on his life. De Quincey was a serious addict for 17 years, but never stopped taking opium completely. *Confessions* was an instant success as a bold new form of "drug literature." To this day, it is considered one of the best and most accurate accounts of the personal experience of drug use. De Quincey's work influenced numerous writers, such as Charles Baudelaire, Elizabeth Barrett Browning, John Keats, and Edgar Allan Poe.

Confessions of an English Opium Eater is a testament to opium's insatiable hold on its victims, even those with such great imaginative faculties:

> If opium-eating be sensual pleasure, and if I am bound to confess that I have indulged in it to an excess, not yet recorded of any other man, it is no less true, that I have struggled against this fascinating enthrallment with a religious zeal, and have, at length, accomplished what I never yet heard attributed to any other man—have untwisted, almost to its final links the accursed chain which fettered me.

THE SMOKING OF OPIUM

For thousands of years, before the advent of heroin or purified morphine (and the abundant consumption of laudanum in the West), opium was primarily consumed by smoking it. Smoking opium requires the habitué to engage in a complex process, which necessitates the utilization of a pipe, a spirit (alcohol) lamp, a large needle, an opium container, a large tray to hold all of the supplies, and perhaps most importantly, an environ in which to smoke, often called an **opium den**.

Traditionally, opium is smoked with a pipe, typically around 20 inches long. Opium pipes are usually made of wood, and the type of wood used often denotes the wealth of the smoker. Poor smokers typically use pipes made from bamboo, while wealthier smokers may have pipes constructed of ebony. About three-quarters down the shaft of the pipe rests the bowl, a hollow structure that can be made of metal, porcelain, or clay, again depending on the quality of the pipe. The hollow pipe is sealed on one end and has an opening on the other, through which the user takes in the smoke.

In addition to the pipe, serious smokers require a host of additional materials used to prepare and smoke opium. These include a container to hold the opium, a needle to clear the bowl opening, a lamp to ignite the opium, and a tray to hold all of the supplies.

Whether or not the opium smoker is wealthy, the actual process of smoking the drug is the same. First, the smoker rolls a pea-shaped ball of opium, which is placed on the end of the needle and cooked in the flame of the lamp until it swells and changes from dark brown to golden. The cooked opium is then placed inside the bowl and is ready to be smoked. The smoker lies on his or her side, holding the pipe so that the bowl opening is right next to the lamp flame. While reclining, the smoker takes long breaths, dragging the smoke into his or her lungs. The serious smoker will prepare several pipes and smoke continually until satisfied.

THE OPIUM DEN

Just as smoking opium typically requires a large setup (a "kit"), for many it also requires a safe haven. This need for a secret place to smoke is responsible for the creation of the opium den.

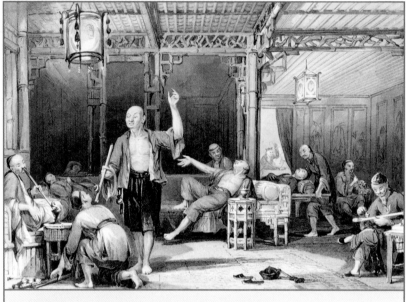

Figure 5.1 Opium den. © Bettmann/CORBIS

Opium dens, like the smoking of opium itself, are often exaggerated and glorified by writers. They are often described as lavish halls with comfortable seating, large tapestries hanging from the walls, and dutiful hostesses waiting to prepare pipes. However, the reality of the dens is often less romantic. Typically, opium dens are crowded, run-down rooms capable of quickly hiding any sign of opium use. The dens are smoky, as they must be sealed lest the onerous smoke escape. For many, though, the experience of smoking opium with others is welcome, regardless of the surroundings.

OTHER WAYS TO SMOKE OPIUM

The method of the opium den constitutes the primary process used by the majority of opium smokers throughout history, but today, smoking opium by other methods is more prevalent in the West. There are other traditional methods of smoking opium in other parts of the world, as well. Opium can be mixed with tobacco and smoked in any number of ways, depending on the individual inclinations of a given population. In Turkey, for example, opium and tobacco were smoked together in tobacco or water pipes. In India, opium was mostly eaten, but when smoked was done so using a hookah (an elongated tobacco pipe) rather than the standard kit. Regardless of how the drug is consumed, it results in both great euphoria and terrible withdrawal.

FROM EUPHORIA TO WITHDRAWAL

Smoking opium has been both lauded and demonized by users, not because of any intrinsic mythical or spiritual attributes accompanying the drug, but as a result of the real physical feelings associated with euphoria and withdrawal. The physical sensations of smoking opium are well documented by those who have used and become addicted to the drug. People who use opium often describe the experience as one of initial relaxation and sleepiness. Opium's most sought after attribute is that, when smoked, it draws the user into a state of complacency where nothing seems to matter and all cares simply float away. Addicts describe an initial calmness that eventually develops into a serene euphoria. Accompanying these feelings, users also describe an initial enhanced mental activity. The effect is likened to the imagination exploding (it is this attribute that leads writers and artists to celebrate opium's seemingly muse-like effects).

Users also describe additional effects, such as an insatiable hunger, especially for sweet foods, and constipation. After a while, users report a lessening of the effects of opium, as the body adapts to its use. Typically, after a few weeks of use, sensations of euphoria are only mild. This adjustment causes the user to increase their level of consumption. Over time, the smoker becomes an addict, and with addiction comes a new range of feelings.

Of all the various concoctions or variations of using opium, from straight morphine to codeine to heroine, the withdrawal experienced from smoking raw opium is probably the least severe, although withdrawal still occurs. While the amount of time necessary before an addiction occurs varies from person to person, all addicts experience feelings of depression and lethargy when not actively using the drug. At first, addiction comes with physical decline in the form of general weakness. As addiction continues, the user will lose concentration, and as a result of constantly suppressing his or her appetite, may begin to appear thinner and eventually emaciated. Long-term addicts experience memory loss and have reported a range of serious medical conditions, such as liver damage, psychosomatic disorders, and lost fertility. For serious addicts, while most bodily functions become depressed, hearing and sight are intensified and often noise and lights become amplified and painful. Some users even report hallucinations.

While not all users become addicts or experience the same intensity of addiction, the effects are real and constitute significant negative health implications. In his 1958 study "Drugs and Mind," Robert S. Ropp provides a concise and descriptive account of opiate withdrawal:

> About twelve hours after the last dose of morphine or heroine the addict begins to grow uneasy. A sense of weakness overcomes him, he yawns, shivers, and sweats all at the same time while a watery discharge pours from his eyes and inside the nose, which he compares to "hot water funning up into the mouth." For a few hours, he falls into an abnormal tossing, restless sleep known among addicts as the yen sleep. On awakening, eighteen to twenty-four hours after his last dose of the drug, the addict begins to enter the lower depths of his personal hell. The yawning may be so violent as to dislocate the jaw, watery mucus pours from the nose and copious tears

from the eyes. The pupils are widely dilated, the hair on the skin stands up, and the skin itself is cold and shows that typical goose flesh which in the parlance of the addict is called "cold turkey," a name also applied to the treatment of addiction by means of abrupt withdrawal.

ANTI-OPIUM CRUSADE

There is little mystery behind the fact that opium, as such an extremely addictive drug, that creates such intense euphoria, became a world commodity when left unregulated. By the late nineteenth century, opium was traded globally on an enormous scale, tantamount to other major products such as coffee and tea. As millions of people became addicts, and the terrible withdrawal effects were increasingly realized, an anti-opium crusade developed in many nations with the goal of eradicating opium altogether.

In the beginning of the crusade, Chinese missionaries, Chinese imperial officers, and British Protestants joined forces to create mass support for global anti-opium regulations. This group, formerly called the Anglo-Oriental Society for the Suppression of the Opium Trade, ultimately succeeded when the British government officially ended India's opium exports in 1906. By 1919, the licit opium trade between China and India was officially over. In the United States, a parallel call for the control of opium emerged and the government responded by banning opium in the Philippines (a U.S. protectorate at the time) by 1908. This ban preceded serious efforts to curb domestic opium use.

For the next several decades, as international laws became tougher and the licit opium trade significantly curtailed, crime syndicates increasingly emerged as the new movers and sellers of opium. Even with harsh new laws, the demand for opium continued, and the only real change was the name of the seller. Nevertheless, by the early twentieth century, the public no longer viewed opium as a gift from the heavens. Instead, the majority regarded it as a most terrible demon.

TREATING OPIUM ADDICTION

Opium has been used as a medicine for hundreds of years, inevitably creating countless addicts. Scientists have conducted a never-ending search for effective cures for opium addiction, morphine addiction (morphinism), and heroin addiction. For most of its history, opium addiction was treated as a disease with no cure, and doctors concerned themselves with treating the symptoms of addiction rather than the root cause. As a result, other opiates were used to lessen the effects of withdrawal. The addict is placed on a regimen of opiates that slowly decrease over time, weaning the addict from his or her addiction. This process of treatment is still used today.

Over the years, scores of seemingly counterintuitive methods have been tried to cure the addict. When morphine was first isolated and synthesized, it was considered to be, and utilized as, a cure for opium addiction. Later, heroin was created, and used as a treatment for morphinism. In the mid-twentieth century, lysergic acid diethylamide (LSD) likewise was tried as a therapy. The sad truth is that even today there is no real cure for any of the various forms of opiate addiction.

Modern therapy uses a drug called methadone. Methadone, discovered in the 1940s, is similar to morphine and heroin as a powerful analgesic. When injected, methadone prevents heroin and morphine from working and lessens the withdrawal effects of both. While also an addictive drug, methadone is used to treat heroin and morphine addiction because it is supposedly easier to quit using. Essentially, an addict on the therapy is given a dose of methadone equivalent to that of their heroin or morphine use. The patient receives lower and lower dosages, until they eventually need no drug at all.

Many addicts, however, report that weaning themselves off of methadone is just as bad as coming off of heroin or morphine addiction. Ultimately, primary treatments for opiate addiction rely on replacing one drug for another and are essentially palliative treatments. The user is never "cured" and will always be tormented by the specter of addiction.

6

The Advance of Heroin

FROM RAW OPIUM TO HEROIN

By the 1800s, opium already had a long, tumultuous history of extensive use. During this time, even with a burgeoning anti-opium movement, scientists convinced of opium's great medicinal potential began to study the drug more closely. Scientists were trying to discover and isolate opium's central chemical, which was unknown at the time. Little did they know that they would find a compound that would far exceed opium in its addictive and destructive potential—heroin.

As scientists began examining the nefarious poppy, they learned how to isolate opium's individual chemical entities. In 1804, a pharmacist from France named Derosyne first isolated what he thought to be the single essence of opium. At the time, it was believed that all of the effects of opium were caused by a single compound. But Derosyne had, in fact, discovered only one of the many chemicals in opium, noscapine.

Just two years later, a pharmacist's assistant from Germany, Friedrich Wilhelm Adam Serturner, made a huge breakthrough. Through his experiments, Serturner realized that while opium was thought to be completely acidic, it contained basic (alkaline) qualities as well. Calling these basic substances "alkaloids," Serturner isolated a pure substance that he believed to be opium's essence. He called this substance "morphium" after the mythical Greek god of sleep, Morpheus. Serturner had discovered morphine, the most powerful compound in opium.

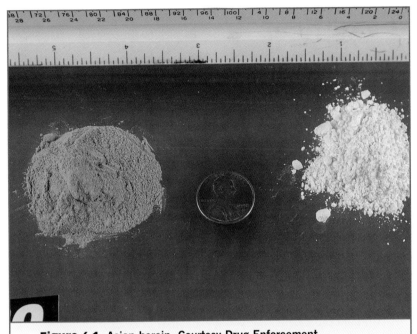

Figure 6.1 Asian heroin. Courtesy Drug Enforcement Administration

Over the following decades, many of the other alkaloids in opium were isolated, including codeine in 1832, thebaine in 1835, and papaverine in 1848. Morphine, however, became increasingly more popular as both a medicinal and recreational product. By the latter half of the eighteenth century, as morphine revealed itself to be a menacing drug creating countless addicts, scientists again examined and manipulated the compound in an effort to find a cure for morphinism. In 1874, pharmacist C. R. Alder Wright stumbled across a new, more powerful formulation of morphine. Through a process of boiling morphine with acetic anhydride, a new chemical called tetra-ethyl morphine was created.

Years later, in 1898, Heinrich Dreser, a chemist working for Bayer Laboratories, conducted a series of clinical tests with the previously discovered tetra-ethyl morphine (now renamed diacetylmorphine). Dreser found that the new compound had incredibly strong pain-relieving qualities. Now officially under the marketing control of Bayer Laboratories, the drug was mass produced and advertised as the new wonder drug. In coining a brand name for the new product, Dreser used the German word *heroisch*, meaning heroic, and called the product **heroin** (Figure 6.1).

HOW HEROIN IS MADE

We have learned about the process of extracting morphine from raw opium. By today's scientific standards, this is a relatively easy process, because morphine is a single chemical

TAPPING THE VEIN

Up until the 1800s, the primary methods of consuming opium were ingesting it or smoking it. But just as opium was examined to find more powerful, concentrated substances, physicians sought new methods of administering drugs that were more effective and had fewer side effects. In the 1830s, physicians began using a medical tool, consisting of a syringe combined with a needle, to inject drugs intravenously. By 1853, the method had been perfected.

At first, the new hypodermic needle was hailed as a better way to administer morphine. The primary advantage of the needle, it was believed, was that it would not create the unwanted addiction associated with imbibing or smoking opium. The rationale was that addiction was associated with hunger or appetite, and because the needle allowed the user to avoid ingesting the drug, no addiction would occur. However, it was soon realized that the hypodermic needle, as a more potent form of drug administration, did not let users escape addiction. In fact, injection of the drug made addiction even more likely.

compound that already exists in the plant. Heroin, while similarly easy to produce, differs from morphine because it is not a natural compound in opium, but a chemical produced by altering extracted morphine.

HOW HEROIN IS USED

While heroin can be smoked and inhaled in its powder form, the primary method of administration is through intravenous injection. To inject heroin, the user mixes the powder with water, heats it, suctions it into a hypodermic needle, and injects it into a muscle or directly into a vein. Once in the body, heroin acts much more rapidly than morphine, crossing the

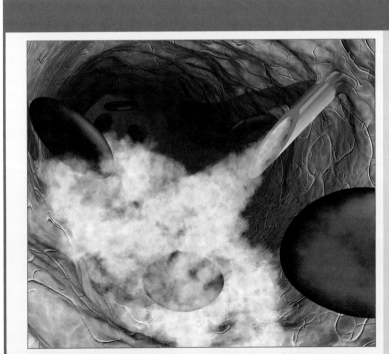

Figure 6.2 Drug injection into a vein. © Roger Harris/Photo Researchers, Inc.

blood/brain barrier 100 times faster. When injected directly into a vein, the effects of heroin can be felt in less than 8 seconds (5–8 minutes when injected into a muscle).

Because both the dangers and addictiveness of heroin are well known, many wonder why users begin to inject heroin at all. While there is no single predominating factor that leads to heroin use, the use of other, less harmful drugs often plays a role. Peer pressure and other psychological factors can also lead to heroin use. Interestingly, users report that the very first experience with heroin is not a pleasant one. The user often feels nauseous and sick after their first use of the drug. Even so, the addictive power of heroin is so strong that many continue to use it, and after several tries the user will experience the drug's sought after effects.

The overall effect that heroin has is to depress the body's central nervous system. However, other short-term effects include a brief euphoria, reduced pain, sedation/drowsiness, reduced anxiety, and reduced respiration. Because of its potent nature, addiction to heroin occurs rapidly. Once addicted, the user craves heroin about five hours after their last injection. The withdrawal symptoms of heroin are also acute and occur about 10 hours after the last use. Withdrawal symptoms progress in intensity and severity over the next three days and only slowly subside after about 10 days. Ultimately, the user is left with a psychological addiction that may take months or even years to overcome.

The user also faces other dangers, especially when injecting heroin, such as possible contraction of human immunodeficiency virus/acquired immunodeficiency syndrome (HIV/AIDS) from sharing needles and death resulting from an overdose of the drug. A heroin overdose occurs as a result of the drug's effect on the respiratory system. When too much of the drug is taken, breathing is slowed to such a point that the user falls into a coma and, in some cases, the user may stop breathing altogether.

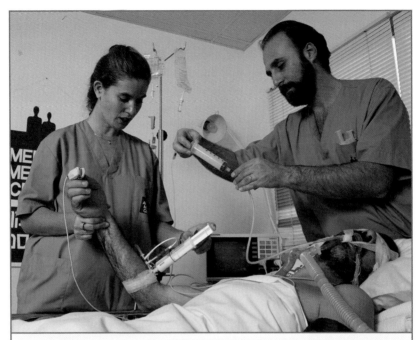

Figure 6.3 Unconscious addict receiving medical treatment.
© Ricki Rosen/CORBIS SABA

HEROIN TRADE EXPANDS

Heroin was at first hailed as a new wonder drug that could effectively reduce coughs and control respiratory problems. Later, although it is much more potent than morphine, heroin was advertised as a cure for morphine addiction. Originally, heroin was distributed in pills and even as cough lozenges. Within just a few years, heroin became a popular drug, widely used throughout the United States and Europe. It did not take long, however, for medical professionals to realize the addictive nature of the drug, and they quickly stopped pronouncing heroin to be a useful drug and began to speak out against its use.

By the turn of the twentieth century, however, it was too late. Even with heroin in disrepute, it had already gained a strong foothold as a profitable worldwide commodity, and its production and trade could not be stopped. Heroin, even more so than opium, was an ideal drug for trade. Heroin, as a white powder, was lighter than opium, much more potent, and much

OXYCONTIN® CRAZE

Recently, many health advocates have become concerned with a prescription drug called OxyContin. Manufactured by Purdue Pharma, OxyContin is the brand name for the drug oxycodone hydrochloride. Concern about this drug is a result of its increasing non-medical abuse. In 2003, for example, the National Survey on Drug Use and Health found that about 2.8 million people older than 12 years of age had used OxyContin at least once non-medically. The problem, perhaps, is that OxyContin is extremely good at doing its job—pain relief. OxyContin is a powerful prescription medication used by millions of people annually to treat severe pain.

Unlike other pain-relievers such as aspirin or Tylenol, which have a limit to the amount of pain relief they can deliver, OxyContin's effectiveness increases in proportion to the amount taken. In other words, after a certain point, adding another aspirin will not do anything more for pain, whereas an increase in OxyContin will keep the patient feeling better and better. Under these circumstances, it is easy to see why the drug lends itself to easy abuse.

But the question remains: if OxyContin is such a great drug, why the concern? It stems from the fact that OxyContin comes from the poppy plant, in the form of the alkaloid thebaine. While less powerful than raw opium, and certainly much less powerful than heroin, thebaine is still an opiate easier to transport secretly. Heroin was also much easier to adulterate, through the addition of other powders, and could be sold at higher price than opium. Once raw opium is obtained, heroin can be cooked up in any small laboratory, anywhere in the world. But this also means that the purity and contents of heroin sold on the street can vary widely.

and thus comes with high addictive potential. As a result, the drug falls under the Schedule II controlled substances section of the U.S. Drug Enforcement Administration (DEA) code, which means that its distribution is more tightly regulated. As a highly effective and useful prescription medication and simultaneously abused drug, OxyContin will likely continue to invite both praise and admonishment.

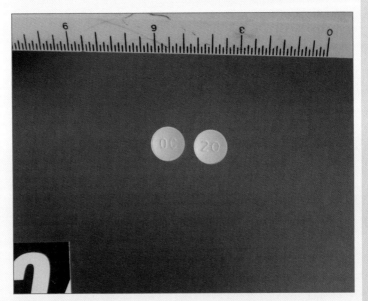

Figure 6.4 OxyContin, 20 milligrams. Courtesy Drug Enforcement Administration

Today, the heroin trade consists of a long distribution chain, with high profits along each link. While the biggest dealers buy bulk quantities of up to 100 kilos from places like Hong Kong and Bangkok, they typically divide up the shipment into small units, or "bags," of 1–10 kilos, which are distributed to small-time dealers for sale to the general public. These small bags can be sold from anywhere between $5 and $100. By the time it hits the streets, the value of heroin grows

THE WORLDWIDE HEROIN TRADE

According to the U.S. National Drug Intelligence Center's *National Drug Threat Assessment 2005* report, heroin is "readily available" in most major cities in the United States. While Chicago, Los Angeles, and New York were designated as the primary distribution centers, Baltimore, Miami, Detroit, Philadelphia, Newark, San Francisco, Seattle, Boston, and Washington, D.C., were also listed as primary centers of heroin distribution. The market for heroin is large, to say the least. In the United States in 2003, for example, more than 310,000 people older than 12 years of age reported some level of heroin use. In 2002, there were 285,667 heroin addict admissions to publicly funded treatment facilities, according to the report.

In 2003, worldwide heroin production was placed at approximately 426.9 metric tons from eight major producing countries, including Mexico, Colombia, Afghanistan, Burma, Laos, Pakistan, Thailand, and Vietnam. It is interesting to note that the production of heroin in Afghanistan dropped significantly in 2001 to just seven tons, after the Taliban government there declared its cultivation and use "un-Islamic" and illegal. However, since then production has rapidly increased to a total of 337 tons, making Afghanistan the current world leader in heroin production.

ten times. A kilo of heroin purchased from Southeast Asia for $100,000 would eventually earn a total of $1 million. According to the U.S. Drug Enforcement Agency, the cost of 1 kilo of heroin from Southeast Asia in 1997 was between $100,000 and $120,000. In general, it takes 10 tons of raw opium to produce one ton of heroin. The lucrative nature of the illicit heroin trade is irresistible for many, and thus it thrives as the main outlet for the production of opium.

Table 6.1 Potential Worldwide Heroin Production, in Metric Tons, 1999–2003

	1999	2000	2001	2002	2003	2004
Mexico	8.8	4.5	10.7	6.8	11.9	NA*
Colombia	8.7	8.7	11.4	8.5	7.8	NA*
Afghanistan	218.0	365.0	7.0	150.0	337.0	582.0
Burma	104.0	103.0	82.0	60.0	46.0	28.0
Laos	13.0	20.0	19.0	17.0	19.0	5.0
Pakistan	4.0	19.0	0.5	0.5	5.2	NA*
Thailand	0.6	0.6	0.6	0.9	NA	NA*
Vietnam	1.0	1.4	1.4	1.0	NA	NA*
Total	358.1	522.2	132.6	244.7	426.9	NA*

Source: CIA Crime and Narcotics Center
* Estimates for 2004 not completed at time of data publication.

Source: National Drug Intelligence Center. National Drug Threat Assessment 2005, Executive Summary. Washington, D.C.: National Drug Intelligence Center, 2005. Available online. URL: http://www.usdoj.gov/ndic/pubs11/13745/heroin.htm. Accessed June 2, 2006.

7

Opium Comes to America

During the nineteenth century heroin was just beginning to enter the world stage, and opium was simultaneously taking root in America. The opium trade in the 1800s was well established and had translated into huge profits at the expense of creating numerous addicts. Up until this point, the use of opium, though technically illegal in China, was primarily concentrated within that area of the world. By the mid-1800s the opium peddled to China by the West would come back with a vengeance. The vehicle for this new infusion of opium at home was industrialization.

By 1850, the United States was becoming an ever-increasing land of prosperity. The rags to riches "American Dream" ideal was in full tilt, and while it was not universal, the dream was true for many. The precipitous forces of industrialization were beginning to flourish, creating new industries that required new work-forces, the California Gold Rush had brought swaths of American frontiersmen to the West coast in the search for unbridled wealth, and the influx of people created a burgeoning railroad industry that soon exploded.

As a result of this new economic activity, America experienced an unprecedented wave of immigration. Many of these immigrants were impoverished and came to America looking for jobs and the promise of a better life. For many poor workers in China, America appeared to be a promised land of opportunity. California became home to masses of Chinese immigrants. The myth of America as a receptacle of wealth is evidenced by the Chinese term for the United States at the time—the "Golden Mountain."

Thousands of Chinese immigrants came to California during the 1850s. More than 20,000 Chinese came to California in 1850; in 1852, 30,000 came from Hong Kong to San Francisco alone. For the most part, the new immigrants worked in newly discovered gold mines or on the railroads. Most immigrants had little or no money, and the majority entered as indentured servants, workers who exchanged their labor for passage into the United States. These immigrants were generally treated poorly and paid pitifully.

IMMIGRANTS AND OPIUM

Chinese immigrants were often blamed for bringing opium to America, but opium had been present in America for some time, both in its raw form and in countless medical concoctions created by patent medicine makers, the unlicensed pharmacists of the day. Nevertheless, the wave of Chinese immigrants, who had used opium in China or picked up the habit in America, enhanced the demand for opium and thus expanded the market.

In response to the intense rigors, harsh conditions, and extensive physical strain of working in the railroad and gold mine industries, many of the immigrants sought the pain-relief and euphoria opium provided. The absence of Chinese women in California resulted in a large male population that often turned to opium as solace for the lack of romantic relations.

Initially, business owners tolerated and even supported the use of opium among their immigrant workers. At the time, opium was still legal in the United States. Manufacturers were happy to produce and deliver the drug, and the government was happy to collect the high taxes garnered from its sale. Furthermore, business owners viewed opium as a source of control. Opium kept the workforce happy, willing and able to continue in what was effectively a slave labor situation.

CHINATOWNS

The extensive Chinese immigration into America, coupled with the racism that Chinese immigrants met when they arrived in America, resulted in the development of distinctly Chinese enclaves in U.S cities. These new neighborhoods, usually situated within larger U.S. cities, were known as Chinatowns. Chinatowns provided a range of necessities to incoming immigrants, including housing and a network of fellow Chinese who could assist in finding gainful employment. But Chinatowns also served another purpose as ready hubs for the distribution of opium. By the 1850s, significant Chinatowns began to appear on America's west coast as laborers searched for work in the gold mines and on the railroads.

Chinatowns were important for the introduction of opium in America. The neighborhoods provided central locations with high demand for the drug. Over the years, countless opium dens began appearing in the various Chinatowns on the west coast of America and Canada. At one point there were more than 300 opium dens in San Francisco alone. As Chinatowns were established across the country, the opium dens followed. By 1876, Chinatown in New York City was firmly established, and opium use spread across the country, moving from Chinatown to Chinatown. While raw opium may have been novel to many Americans of the day, its constituents were certainly not. Opium had already pervaded the homes of many Americans through the patent medicine men.

THE PATENT MEDICINE MAKERS

In the 1800s, there were no large-scale pharmaceutical manufacturers, no carefully tested safe and effective medicines, and no regulatory body (such as the U.S. Food and Drug Administration) to make sure that medicines were safe to use and actually worked. Instead, there were the patent medicine makers, which were unregulated small-time drug manufacturers. The profession of patent medicine making, often referred to as quackery, resulted in the proliferation of thousands of untested medications, called nostrums, combining all kinds of natural products and drugs.

Many of these nostrums were advertised to cure a myriad of diseases, but probably failed to cure any. However, they certainly created countless alcoholics and morphine addicts. By the early 1900s, concern regarding patent medicines was on the rise and the medical profession soon formally discredited their production. These measures unfortunately came too late to curb the infiltration of opium into American society.

INTERNATIONAL CONTROLS ON OPIUM

Beginning in the early twentieth century, more and more people realized the dangerous nature of opium and its derivatives, and a worldwide effort was established to try to control the growing and selling of opium. The first attempt came in 1909 when the International Opium Commission convened for the first time. The commission was the first international congress on opium and its alkaloids. While only 13 nations attended and the actual results were minor, the meeting was significant because it put opium on the map as a worldwide problem.

The next major convention on opium occurred in 1911 in the Netherlands. A declaration was made at the 1911 convention which advocated all nations to institute domestic opium laws. However, agreements made at the convention were meaningless because individual nations ultimately ignored the statutes. Time and time again, international efforts to control opium consumption were curbed by vested interests. The opium trade was critical to many countries' economies, and the tax revenues were too substantial for many governments to want to effect any change.

While some small strides were made during this time, the advance of World War I pushed aside any substantial legislative action. By the war's end, through the auspices of the newly created League of Nations, a new effort was made. In 1921, the

NEFARIOUS NOSTRUMS

The great majority of medicines produced by the early independent manufacturer contained alcohol, morphine, or even heroin. Moreover, many of these patent medicines were targeted at children: Soothing Baby Syrup, for example, was advertised as way to stop babies from crying; with morphine as its primary constituent, it was effective. Kopp's Baby Friend, which was advertised as a perfect way to calm down babies, was essentially sweetened water and morphine. Other popular nostrums included Lydia E. Pinkman's Vegetable Compound and Dr. Hostetter's Stomach Bitters. As with many medicines of the time, the principal ingredient in these mixtures (20 percent and 44 percent, respectively), was alcohol.

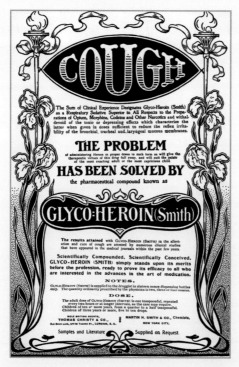

Figure 7.1 Heroin cough syrup. © Bettmann/CORBIS

League set up an Advisory Committee on the Traffic of Opium and Other Dangerous Drugs, with the task of defining the scope of the opium trade and recording statistical information. By 1925, the League convened the Geneva Conference, which began a more intense period of international controls on opium.

While there were still many disputes between individual nations over the terms of opium production and distribution, international action finally proved effective, achieving an 80 percent reduction in worldwide opium production, from 42,000 tons in 1906 to 16,000 tons by 1934. Over the next several decades, international oversight continued, at times lulling (particularly during World War II), but at other times booming, especially after the creation of the United Nations following World War II. However, total control over opium has never been achieved, and illegal opium trade continues to this day. One reason it is so difficult to control opium production is that its cultivation is necessary to supply the lawful pharmaceutical industry.

8

Modern Opiate-Based Medicines

There are many legal medicines that use opiates or opiate-like substances. Most of the opiate-based medicines used today are not made from natural opiates, but are either synthetic or semi-synthetic. Synthetic opiate drugs are not actually opiates at all; they are merely different chemicals that act like opiates. Semi-synthetics are those drugs that involve changing the chemical structure of a natural opiate. An example of this is heroin, which is a human-made variation of morphine. Morphine and codeine are the principal natural opiates used as medicines and what follows are descriptions of the other most frequently used opiate-based medicines.

CODEINE

Codeine is a natural alkaloid found in the opium plant. As a pharmaceutical, codeine is used as an analgesic, antitussive, and antidiarrheal. Codeine is also commonly combined with other cough suppressants as well as with aspirin and ibuprofen. In the United States, codeine is a Schedule III controlled substance, which means that its distribution is more tightly regulated than unscheduled drugs. Codeine has pain-relieving qualities principally because, once in the body, about 10 percent of codeine turns into morphine. This conversion occurs in the liver, where an enzyme changes codeine's chemical structure. The potential side effects of codeine include itching, vomiting, nausea, drowsiness, dry mouth, miosis, orthostatic hypotension, constipation, and urinary retention. The most serious side effect, however, is respiratory depression, which is potentially fatal. Codeine is a popular pharmaceutical, and it is abused all over the world. In the United States, people often take much higher than recommended doses of codeine to experience its opioid effects.

DIHYDROCODEINE

Related to codeine, **dihydrocodeine** is a rather weak analgesic, usually combined with other drugs and used as a headache suppressant. It is often, however, prescribed for postoperative pain, dyspnea, and as an antitussive. Dihydrocodeine is twice as potent as codeine.

FENTANYL

Fentanyl is a semi-synthetic opioid. It is a much more powerful version of morphine. Fentanyl is used during surgery as an anesthetic and is extremely dangerous when taken in a nonmedical context. First created in Belgium in the 1950s, fentanyl is 80 times more powerful than morphine. Due to its strength, fentanyl is listed as a Schedule I narcotic in the United States. Even though this very powerful pharmaceutical is extremely dangerous, it has been used illicitly at least since the mid-1970s. The various forms of fentanyl can be hundreds of times more powerful than heroin and its effects are indistinguishable. On the street, fentanyl is known as "china white."

HYDROCODONE

Hydrocodone is a widely prescribed (and abused) pharmaceutical designed as a pain-reliever. The drug works by converting into a form of morphine once it enters the body. Hydrocodone can be derived from either codeine or thebaine and is three times more powerful than codeine. Hydrocodone has various trade names,

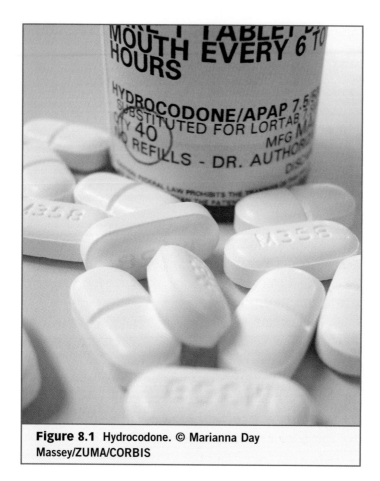

Figure 8.1 Hydrocodone. © Marianna Day
Massey/ZUMA/CORBIS

including Anexsia®, Dicodid®, Hycodan®, Hycomine®, Lorcet®, Lortab®, Norco®, Tussionex®, and the most popular, Vicodin®.

HYDROMORPHONE

Hydromorphone is a pharmaceutical product used to combat severe pain. It is a powerful semi-synthetic opioid that is 10 times more powerful than morphine.

MEPERIDINE

Also known as pethidine, **meperidine** is a synthetic opioid that is often used in place of morphine to treat pain. Meperidine has various trade names, including isonipecaine, lidol, peridine, pethanol, piridosal, Algil®, Alodan, Demerol®, Dispadol, Dolantin, Dolosal®, and Mefedina. Meperidine is sometimes preferred because its side effects, such as constipation and muscle spasm, are not as strong as those produced by morphine. Meperidine has negative interactions with various other medicines, including muscle relaxants, benzodiazepines, antidepressants, and alcohol. The adverse effects of meperidine include dizziness, possible unconsciousness, swelling of the lips, tongue, or face, seizures, clammy skin, and asthma.

METHADONE

Methadone hydrochloride is a synthetic opioid that is commonly used today to treat heroin addicts. First synthesized in 1937, methadone is chemically different from morphine and heroin, but works similarly in the body. Originally known as Dolophine®, methadone is made today by a host of pharmaceutical companies and is used in drug detoxification programs. It is useful for this purpose because it metabolizes at a slower rate than morphine or heroin. Methedone is therefore longer-lasting than other opioids, but has fewer withdrawal symptoms. Many heroin addicts, however, report that it is even harder to quit taking methadone than it is to stop using heroin.

OXYCODONE

Derived from the alkaloid thebaine, **oxycodone** is a highly effective pain-reliever and prescribed to postsurgical patients, cancer patients, and others with severe pain. Oxycodone is sold under various trade names in combination with aspirin, including Percodan®, Endodan, and Roxipirin; with acetaminophen it is marketed as Percocet®, Endocet, and Roxicet. Oxycodone is also the main ingredient in OxyContin. The most frequent side effect of oxycodone is constipation, but naseua is also common. Oxycodone is highly abused in the United States.

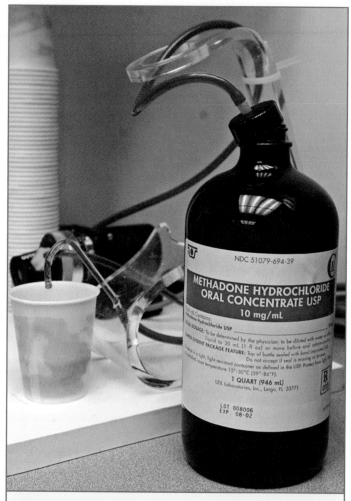

Figure 8.2 Methadone dispenser. © AP/Wide World Photos

PROPOXYPHENE

Propoxyphene is a synthetic opioid that is similar to methadone but much less potent. Propoxyphene is the active ingredient in the pharmaceutical products Darvon-N® and Darvocet-N. It is used by some physicians to treat severe pain and coughs but is hotly debated as a useful medication. Many doctors refuse to prescribe the drug because of its highly addictive nature.

Table 8.1 Common Pharmaceuticals Containing Opiates

Generic Name	Common Brand Name
Codeine	Tylenol® III
Dihydrocodeine	Synalgos® DC
Fentanyl	Duragesic®
Hydrocodone	Vicodin®
Hydromorphine	Dilaudid®
Meperidine	Demerol®
Methadone	Dolophine®
Oxycodone	Percocet®
Oxymorphone	Numorphan®
Propoxyphene	Darvon®

Adapted from Moraes, Francis, and Debra Moraes. *Opium.* Oakland, Calif.: Ronin Publishing, 2003, p. 125.

9

The Opium Trade Today

With all of the various forms that opiates take today, both legal and illicit, it is not surprising that the illegal trade continues to flourish, even in the face of strict international controls on opium. The fact that there are so many legitimate pharmaceutical products based on opium makes controlling opium production extremely difficult. The real need for the chemicals in opium that are used to create medicines inevitably allows for some of that opium to be moved through clandestine channels. Unfortunately, the proportion of opium production relegated to illegal ends far outweighs that of necessary opium production.

THE NEW OPIUM TRADE

The creation of tougher national and international laws in the late twentieth century has resulted in a slight transformation of the opium trade. Laws have become stricter and limited success has been made in raising public awareness concerning the dangerous nature of opium and its constituents. The trade has not stopped, however; it has only changed hands. In the past, the demand for opium created a large and complex distribution chain, complete with opium producers, suppliers, manufacturers, distributors, and consumers. Today, that trade, while now primarily in the form of nonmedical pharmaceutical use and heroin, is equally complex and perhaps even more profitable than ever.

The illicit trade of opium is maintained today by a vast network of producers and traffickers who employ seemingly endless tactics to smuggle the product into nations around the world. The demand for opium remains—it is only the legality of the trade that has adjusted. Most nations today have laws banning the recreational use of opium and its constituents, as well as a system for controlling their use, so illegal drug traders have adjusted their efforts to exploit the weaknesses of the system.

Traffickers typically buy opium from both legal and illegal producers. Lawful producers, growing opium legitimately for the pharmaceutical industry, often earn greater income from the opium they sell on the side to black market traffickers. Some nations have lax laws pertaining to opium production, providing ample opium resources to meet the worldwide demand. Traffickers sell to countries where opium is legal, but the greatest profits come from smuggling and selling the drug in countries where it is illegal and the demand high, such as the United States.

It is estimated that for every ounce of opium going to pharmaceutical companies and the production of medicines, 10 ounces go directly to the illicit market. In other words, 90 percent of all opium production is directed toward illegal markets. The transport of opium has changed greatly over the years, but the ingenuity of smugglers has remained a constant.

SMUGGLING OPIUM

For much of the twentieth century, and continuing today, the primary method of smuggling opium has been through cargo ships. Ships carrying hidden or camouflaged opium often pass through border inspections. Some shipments of opium are discovered and confiscated by authorities, but with hundreds of thousands of ships carrying millions of products across the globe, the possibility of locating all illegal opium shipments is very low. Smugglers are extremely clever in devising ways to conceal their shipments, whether raw opium, heroin, or some other form. Martin Booth, in *Opium: A History*, provides an excellent summary of just a few of the known smuggling tactics:

> Cargoes provided good camouflage: opium or heroin has appeared, amongst many others, in the cargoes of dried shrimps, soap (with opium cakes looking like the bars of soap), in duck egg shells packed alongside real eggs, in Bologna sausage skins, in barrels of cement, in loaves of bread and in tins marked pickled cabbage. . . . A famous instance of the smugglers' artifice concerned opium from Hong Kong entering North America inside the horns of imported cattle.

There are countless ways for smugglers to conceal their shipments, and often a ship's captain and crew are not even aware that they are transporting the product. In addition, traffickers send their shipments through several ports to confuse customs officials and blur the product's country of origin. By the time the drug reaches its destination, even if it is discovered, the traffickers usually remain unknown.

In the latter half of the twentieth century, new avenues of illicit drug distribution emerged, along with new ways to transport opium, emerged. As a result of World War II, which periodically cut off the opium trade, Mexico grew in stature as a primary mover of opium to the United States. It was during this time that drugs were first smuggled by aircraft. The huge border shared by Mexico and the United States, especially the long banks of the Rio Grande River, provides ample sites to move drugs between the countries. To this day, border smuggling remains one of the primary methods of shipping illegal drugs into the United States.

THE "MULES"

Shipping opium remains the primary method of drug trafficking, but the task of transporting opium and heroin is also accomplished on a person-by-person basis. These couriers of

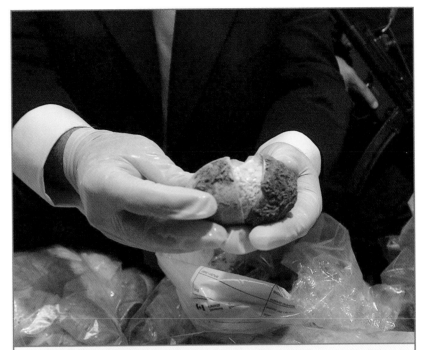

Figure 9.1 Heroin smuggled inside fake duck eggs.
© Reuters/CORBIS

opium, or "**mules**" as they are colloquially known, carry drugs across borders at great personal risk. Typically, the mule is poor and convinced to smuggle drugs in exchange for a small fee, but tourists and diplomatic personnel have also been discovered as drug transporters. The mules who actually carry the drugs into foreign countries are almost never significant persons within the drug distribution chain. These individuals often have little, and usually no, knowledge of the drug dealer they're working for. This method of drug transport is one of many that allows the wealthy drug lords to stay in business, operating in the shadows of international trade.

While many mules simply attempt to carry opium and its constituents in their baggage, a more gruesome and dangerous practice known as "stuffing" or "swallowing" is also prevalent.

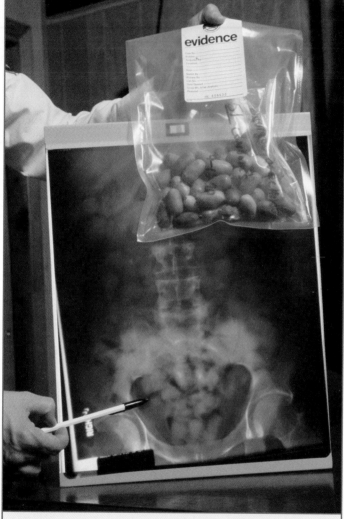

Figure 9.2 X-ray of a drug smuggler's stomach.
© Jacques M. Chenet/CORBIS

This method requires the mule to ingest or insert the drug into his or her body by various means, either through the mouth, vagina, or anus, before traveling across an international border. The drugs are usually wrapped in small rubber containers or satchels (such as condoms and rubber gloves tied with dental floss), held during transport, and passed out of the body in the new country. This practice achieves high success rates because only an X-ray can detect the smuggled product. However, it is extremely dangerous, for if even a single ingested packet tears, the carrier will die of an overdose.

In spite of all of the dangers associated with opium trafficking—the heavy fines, imprisonment, and possible death for the couriers—the potential profits of the trade remain too high to resist. As a result, the transport of opium remains a reality. It flows across borders in quantities equal to some legal products and its trade is maintained by huge networks of people, all taking a piece of the profits. The top drug lords operate with a business savvy equivalent to the chief executive officers (CEOs) of the largest corporations, adjusting to changing markets and even planning for and estimating the loss of some product at customs points. These losses, however, pose little threat to the overall business, which is often so diversified that the discovery of a single shipment does nothing to affect the trade. The drug lords are also extremely wealthy and capable of hiring first-rate lawyers and paying out bribes to many officials.

OPIUM AND THE MOB

The market for opium, and especially heroin, has remained relatively unchanged through the twentieth century, but the various networks and connections through which opium enters the country have changed. In the beginning of the 1900s, when opium was still not well regulated and therefore easy to acquire, there was no need for underground networks to distribute the product. When the Harrison Narcotics Act in 1914 created tight regulations for opium distribution, getting opium became much harder and as a result the black market for opium expanded.

This growing underground market required a network to import the illegal substance and get it to the vast numbers of addicts. This job was initially taken up by various Jewish gangsters in large U.S. cities such as New York. Gangsters such as Benjamin "Bugsy" Siegel, Waxey Gordon, and Louis Buchalter initially controlled the trade, obtaining opium (primarily in the form of heroin) from China, France, and the Middle East. At the same time, the infamous Italian Mafia was gaining strength as thousands of Italian immigrants entered the country. Throughout the 1920s, the mob established itself and gained incredible wealth through the organization and sale of alcohol during prohibition. Clandestine operations during prohibition provided the mob with the experience it needed to take over the heroin syndicate.

The mob was initially hesitant to enter the drug trade, as trafficking was seen as morally reprehensible. However, when prohibition ended and the criminals needed a new source of income, opium became too irresistible. The new leaders of the underworld developed the heroin trade to an extent never before seen in the United States. Through its contacts in Italy, the mob (under the auspices of boss Charles "Lucky" Luciano) created an international chain of distribution. Opium was produced and purchased in Turkey and the larger "Golden Crescent," sent through France, and then shipped to the United States. This "French Connection" was responsible for the great proportion of heroin sold in America from the 1940s through the 1970s.

In the 1970s, President Nixon's "war on drugs," coupled with increasing regulation of opium production in the Golden Crescent (Turkey, Afghanistan, and Pakistan), reduced the overall trade. However, the trade was never wiped out completely, and much of the production has since shifted to Southeast Asia and then back to the Golden Crescent. The opium trade has continued to change and evolve, and will most likely continue to do so for the foreseeable future.

THE GLOBALIZATION OF OPIUM

The global opium trade of the last 30 or so years is best described as a seesaw, waxing and waning in the changing world. When the production of opium falls in one area, it increases in another. During the late 1970s and early 1980s, overall American opium consumption dropped as a result of several factors. A drought in Southeast Asia combined with the Russian invasion of Afghanistan in 1979 led to temporarily decreased production. In the changeable drug culture of America, the shortage of one drug often parallels an increased demand for another. When less opium was available and heroin prices rose, the U.S. experienced an upsurge in cocaine use and addictions.

Continuing the anti-drug platform of the Nixon era, Ronald Reagan's war on drugs battled American narcotics consumption with mixed results. American efforts to control drug use by going after its sources of production increased the overall production and resilience of the trade. When governments concentrated regulatory efforts on specific areas, such as Colombia or Afghanistan, opium production simply shifted to new areas (especially Southeast Asia) creating a larger global area of opium production. Southeast Asia was, as a result, responsible for supplying as much as 80 percent of America's heroin market in the late 1980s and early 1990s. During this period the number of heroin addicts in America increased dramatically.

With a strong production zone in Southeast Asia and the end of hostilities between Russia and Afghanistan, the world supply of opium increased markedly throughout the 1990s. Afghani warlords in the 1990s absorbed greater control over large regions of the country and thus over the production of opium, causing an increase in that production. Afghanistan's production of opium dropped significantly in 2001 after the Taliban outlawed its use and cultivation. However, following the expulsion of the Taliban later that year, production regained its strength and is currently responsible for more than 75 percent of the world's opium supply.

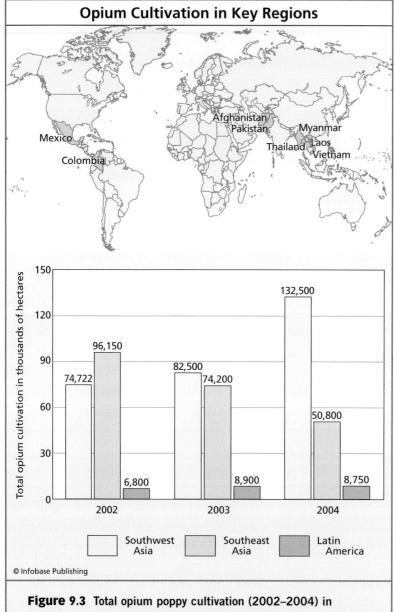

Figure 9.3 Total opium poppy cultivation (2002–2004) in Southwest Asia, Southeast Asia, and Latin America (in hectares).

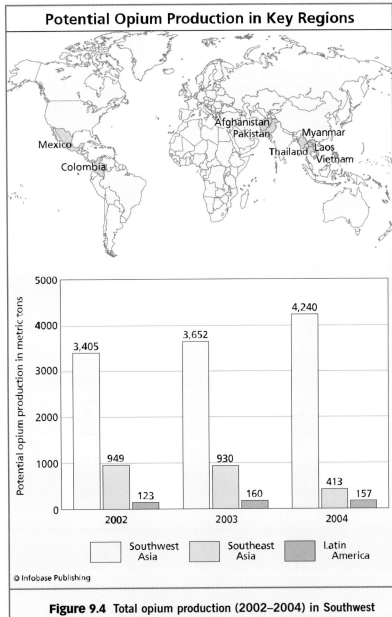

Figure 9.4 Total opium production (2002–2004) in Southwest Asia, Southwest Asia, and Latin America (in metric tons).

AFGHANISTAN:
OPIUM AS A WAY OF LIFE

Is growing opium a crime, or is it a legitimate way of life? For many, societal forces determine which crops will be produced. Farmers grow crops that can earn them enough money to support their families. In 1972, the U.S. government estimated that the average farmer in Afghanistan could earn $300–$360 per hectare from growing poppies for opium. In comparison, the same farmer could earn only $175 per hectare from a fruit crop. Since that time, little has changed. As Amy Waldman of the New York Times recently reported, growing opium is more than an illegal trade—it is a way of life and the road to prosperity for many:

> Across Afghanistan, opium cultivation is surging, defying all efforts of the Afghan government and international officials to stop it. Officials are predicting that land under poppy cultivation will rise by 30% or more this year, possibly yielding a record crop. Last year the country produced almost 4,000 tons—three-fourths of the world's opium—in 28 of its 32 provinces. The trade generated $1 billion for farmers and $1.3 billion for traffickers, according to the United Nations, more than half of Afghanistan's national income. . . .

Source: Waldman, Amy. "Afghan Route to Prosperity: Grow Poppies." *New York Times* (April 10, 2004).

10

Teenage Trends and Attitudes

The majority of the available information supports the notion that teenage use of opium and its derivatives is declining. The use of raw opium in the United States is extremely limited, mostly because little or none is available. Most opium today is used to produce other drugs like heroin and the wide range of prescription drugs that are used in both medicinal and abusive ways. While overall use of heroin is quite small among the teenage population, the abuse of prescription medications that contain opium is on the rise.

Reliable figures on teenage use of drugs have been officially kept since 1975, with the establishment of the Monitoring the Future Survey (MTF). The MTF is a continuing study conducted by the University of Michigan's Institute for Social Research and funded by the National Institute on Drug Abuse (NIDA). The survey collects data from eighth, tenth, and twelfth graders, on both the perceptions and the actual use of drugs over 30-day, annual, and lifetime periods.

According to the MTF, the use of heroin among these students was relatively small. In these grades, approximately 1.5 percent of students had ever tried heroin, and only 0.5 percent reported using heroin in the last 30 days (Table 10.1).

While the use of pure heroin among teens was found to be small, and unchanged from 2003 to 2004, the study did indicate that teens' perception of heroin as a dangerous substance has markedly declined. An additional and more detailed study conducted by the Community Epidemiological Work Group (a subset of the MTF

Table 10.1 Heroin Use by Students, 2004

	8th Graders	10th Graders	12th Graders
Lifetime*	1.6%	1.5%	1.5%
Annual	1.0%	0.9%	0.9%
30-Day	0.5%	0.5%	0.5%

* "Lifetime" refers to use at any point within the respondent's lifetime.
Source: National Survery on Drug Use and Health

study group) found that the use of heroin was higher in the northeastern, north-central, mid-Atlantic, and northwestern parts of the country, where the drug is more readily available. The study also found that heroin use was more frequent in large cities, with the highest incidence of heroin/opium-related deaths in 2002 occurring in Detroit (464) and Philadelphia (111). In the same year, it was found that, nationwide, 13,000 teens between the ages of 12 and 17 had used heroin at least once in the past year. This group made up a relatively small percentage of the total population using heroin that year (404,000).

While the overall use of opium in heroin form among teens is small, the figures are misleading in that they do not represent the full range of drugs containing opiates that are used by teens. A good example of this is MDMA, or as it is more commonly known, ecstasy. Ecstasy, one of a group of drugs categorized as "club drugs" due to their common use in dance club and night club settings, is often laced or mixed with heroin. Because ecstasy comes in pill form, users are often unaware of its actual contents. The use of ecstasy among teens is greater than that of pure heroin. In 2004, 7.5 percent of twelfth graders had reported taking ecstasy at least once, 4 percent had taken it in the last year, and 1.2 percent reported use in the previous 30 days. When considering the level of opium use among teens, it is important to consider more than just raw opium or pure heroin. Teen use of opium becomes even more complex when prescription drugs are added to the mix.

TEEN USE OF PRESCRIPTION DRUGS

As discussed earlier, many of the alkaloids found in the opium plant are used as legitimate medical substances. These drugs, when used appropriately and under the supervision of a medical professional, can be extremely effective medicines. Much of the use of these drugs is, however, actually abuse. The misuse and abuse of prescription drugs is a growing problem among the general population as well as teenagers. According to one study, conducted by the Substance Abuse and Mental Health Services Administration (SAMHSA), 14 percent of teens ages 12–17 reported having abused a prescription medication at least once. Prescription drugs, located in medicine cabinets in the home, are abused by teens because of the accessibility. The abuse of prescription drugs among Americans is second only to the use of marijuana.

An important distinction should be made concerning the difference between the misuse of a drug and abuse of a drug. Misusing a drug occurs when a person with a valid prescription does not follow the instructions for the medicine's proper use. If a patient decided to take three pills in a day when the prescription specifically called for only two pills to be taken, that patient would be misusing the drug. Often, patients believe that more of a medicine will make it work better, but drugs are designed for very specific administration and simply taking more of a drug will not make it more effective. Abuse, on the other hand, refers to the intentional consumption of a prescription medication for some purpose other than what the medicine is indicated for. Abuse is frequent in the case of prescription drugs containing opiates, because abusers seek the medicine's euphoric and pain-relieving effects.

There are three main classes of prescription drugs that are abused: opioids, central nervous system depressants, and stimulants. Opioids are legally used as presurgical medicines or for their pain-relieving qualities, but they are rampantly abused by all sectors of the population. Among the opioids commonly abused are codeine, oxycodone, and hydrocodone (Table 10.2). Use of these drugs remains high among teens. According to the 2003 MTF study, 9.3 percent of high school seniors had used hydrocodone (Vicodin) in the past year. These medications are often taken in addition to other drugs, increasing their effects. Opioids should never be used in combination with alcohol, antihistamines, barbiturates, or benzodiazepines. The greatest concern is that all of these drugs depress the respiratory system. When too many or too much is taken, the possibility of extremely slowed breathing—and even death—becomes much greater.

DRUG TESTING

Testing for drugs is complex and costly. Testing specifically for opiates is especially difficult because the many forms of the drug require individualized testing. In general, testing sites follow the government guidelines designed by NIDA and SAMHSA. The guidelines list five drug categories typically subject to a drug test. The categories are called the NIDA 5, and include: cannabinoids (marijuana, hash), cocaine, amphetamines, opiates (heroin, opium, codeine, and morphine), and phencyclidine (PCP). Testing for the abuse of prescription drugs such as hydrocodone, methadone, or propoxyphene (Darvon) often requires additional exams.

Currently, the available testing methods include urine, blood, hair, saliva, and sweat. The most common of these is the urine test, which is the least invasive and least expensive. Although it is the least expensive of the methods, a urine test might nevertheless cost anywhere from $7–$50. The most accurate tests are blood tests, but these are significantly more expensive and much more invasive as well. Once a sample is taken in any of these forms, there are

Table 10.2 Commonly Abused Prescription Drugs Containing Opium

Substance	Commercial and Street Names	DEA Schedule and Route of Administration	Intoxication Effects and Potential Health Consequences
Codeine	Empirin with Codeine, Fiorinal with Codeine, Robitussin AOC, Tylenol with Codeine; Captain Cody, Cody, schoolboy	II, III, IV; Injected, Swallowed	Drowsiness/respiratory depression and arrest, nausea, confusion, constipation, sedation, unconsciousness, coma, tolerance, addiction
Fetanyl	Actiq, Duragesic, Sublimaze; Apache, China girl, China white, Dance fever, friend, goodfella, jack-pot, murder 8, TNT, tango and cash	II; Injected, Smoked, Snorted	
Morphine	Raxanol, Duramorph; M, Miss Emma, Monkey, White stuff	II, III; Injected, Swallowed, Smoked	
Opium	Laudanum, paregoric; Big O, black stuff, black gum, hop	II, III, V; Swallowed, Smoked	
Other opioid pain-relievers (oxycodone, meperidine, hydromor-phone, hydrocodone, propoxyphene)	Tylox, OxyContin, Percodan, Percocet; Oxy 80s, Oxycotton, Oxycet, hillbilly heroin, percs, Demerol, meperidine hydrochloride; demmies, pain killer, Diaudid; Juice, dillies Vicodin, Lortab, Lorcet; Darvon, Dorvocet	II, III, IV; Swallowed, Injected, Suppositories, Chewed, Crushed, Snorted	

Adapted from National Institute on Drug Abuse. "Information on Drugs of Abuse—Prescription Drug Abuse Chart." Available on the Internet: http://www.drugabuse.gov/DrugPages/PrescripDrugsChart.html.

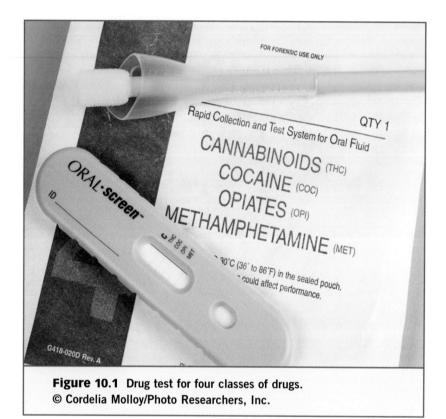

Figure 10.1 Drug test for four classes of drugs.
© Cordelia Molloy/Photo Researchers, Inc.

essentially three options of analysis: gas chromatography, mass spectrometry, and immunoassay (Figures 10.1–10.3).

GAS CHROMATOGRAPHY

First used for drug testing in 1983, gas chromatography is one of the most common methods of drug detection. The gas chromatography machine is able to analyze both urine and blood samples. The sample is first inserted into the machine and vaporized (turned into a gas). As it vaporizes, different metabolites within the sample vaporize at different times, called retention times. The time differences are recorded and analyzed by the machine, which is preprogrammed to recognize the retention times of prohibited drugs.

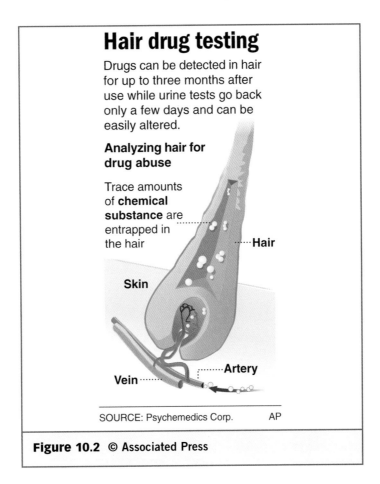

Hair drug testing

Drugs can be detected in hair for up to three months after use while urine tests go back only a few days and can be easily altered.

Analyzing hair for drug abuse

Trace amounts of **chemical substance** are entrapped in the hair

Hair

Skin

Artery

Vein

SOURCE: Psychemedics Corp.   AP

Figure 10.2 © Associated Press

MASS SPECTROMETRY

Along with gas chromatography, mass spectrometry is another of the common ways to detect the presence of prohibited drugs. Mass spectrometry is similar to gas chromatography in that the sample is transferred to a gaseous state and then analyzed. The difference is that a mass spectrometer uses an electron beam to separate the sample into its different ions according to their mass. The machine is able to separate all of the ions into groups and measure their concentrations. The metabolites for many drugs leave their own unique signature. The machine then

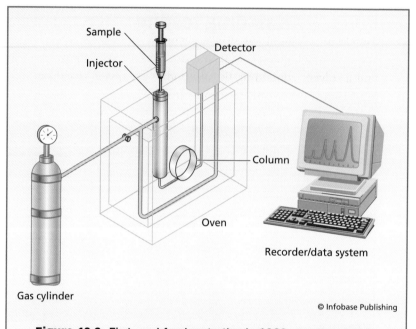

Sample

Injector

Detector

Column

Oven

Recorder/data system

Gas cylinder

© Infobase Publishing

Figure 10.3 First used for drug testing in 1983, gas chromatography is one of the most common methods of drug detection. The gas chromatography machine is able to analyze both urine and blood samples. The sample is first inserted into the machine and vaporized (turned into a gas). As it vaporizes, different metabolites within the sample vaporize at different times, called retention times. The time differences are recorded and analyzed by the machine, which is preprogrammed to recognize the retention times of prohibited drugs.

analyzes the picture created by the electron beam and uses that to identify specific drugs. Typically, a sample is first run through the gas chromatography phase and, if found to contain illicit drugs, it is then run through the mass spectrometer for absolute confirmation.

IMMUNOASSAYS

Immunoassays are another way to detect foreign substances in urine samples. Immunoassays involve the use of antibodies, proteins that can recognize and bind to a specific substance. To test for illegal opiate drugs, scientists find antibodies for the metabolite traces left in the urine by drugs. The urine and a solvent containing the antibodies are mixed together. Scientists are then able to deduce if a drug is present by the reaction between the two substances. Immunochemical assays are common in all kinds of scientific research and are very accurate. While immunoassays are thought to be less desirable than the other analyses, they are typically the first drug testing option used for opium. If an immunoassay results in a positive reading, a further gas chromatography/mass spectrometry analysis may be done to obtain much greater accuracy.

POPULAR CULTURE: MUSICIANS AND HEROIN

With an ethos of "drugs, sex, and rock 'n' roll," the music industry has seen heroin claim many lives over the years. Heroin, specifically, has been the cause of many needless deaths of musicians both young and old, and of all types of music. Below are just of few of the lives taken by heroin.

Kurt Cobain, Nirvana (drug-related suicide, exact cause still debated)

Shannon Hoon, Blind Melon

Janis Joplin

Jonathan Melvoin, Smashing Pumpkins

Jim Morrison, The Doors (exact cause of death still disputed)

Bradley Nowell, Sublime

Sid Vicious, Sex Pistols

DRUG SENSITIVITY AND DETECTION PERIOD

Every drug has its own level of sensitivity, as well as an individual period of detection. Drug sensitivity refers to the amount of drug needed in a drug test sample to consider it a positive result. The detection period is the amount of time within which the test can detect the use of a drug. This amount of time differs, depending on the type of sample—urine, blood, or other. Both an immunoassay and a gas chromatography/mass spectrometry analysis require a sensitivity of 2000 ng/mL (nanogram per milliliter). To help put that sensitivity into perspective, a can of soda contains 355 milliliters, and each milliliter of water has a mass of one billion nanograms. Needless to say, drug tests are capable of detecting very small amounts of a drug.

As previously mentioned, the detection period for a drug depends on a number of factors, including the type of opiate, the type of sample, the frequency of drug use, metabolic rate, age, body mass, drug tolerance, and overall health. Generally speaking opium can be detected for 5–7 days after its use. Other opiates such as heroin and codeine have significantly shorter detection periods (Table 10.3).

Table 10.3 Detection Periods for Opiates

Substance	Blood	Saliva	Sweat	Urine	Hair
Codeine/ Morpine	Unknown	7–21 hours	Unknown	2–4 days	Up to 90 days
Heroin	24–48 hours	Unknown	Unknown	8 hours	Up to 90 days
Opium	5–7 days	5-7 days	Unknown	5–7 days	90–120 days

Adapted from *Vaults of Erowid.* "Drug Testing Basics." Available on the Internet: www.erowid.org/psychoactives/testing/testing_info1.shtml.

Opium and the Law

THE HISTORY OF DRUG CONTROL

Unlike the history of opium use, the history of drug control is comparatively short. In the United States, drug control dates back to the 1840s, when the National Drug Import Law was passed by Congress to ensure that imported drugs were properly labeled. Before this, drugs were totally unregulated by the U.S. government, and there were no established definitions for prescription and nonprescription drugs, narcotics, or drug abuse. There were no laws requiring the manufacturers of drugs to report the quantity and distribution of drugs produced. Manufacturers were not required to conduct tests to make sure that drugs were safe, or carry out clinical trials to prove a drug's effectiveness. In fact, until the 1906 Pure Food and Drug Act, anyone could make or take a concoction or sell any drug to anyone without fear or influence of any government agency. The world we live in today is very different, because drug policies, agencies, and laws have continually grown and evolved. Here are a few of the highlights:

1906—Pure Food and Drug Act: Arguably the most important piece of food and drug legislation in American history, the 1906 act defined both *drug* and *misbranding* and was designed to eliminate false claims. The act led directly to the creation of the Food and Drug Administration (FDA).

1912—Shirley Amendment: Soon after the 1906 act, it was realized that there were innumerable violations that needed attention. The Shirley Amendment was the first attempt by the government to remove fraudulent drugs (drugs that did not do what they claimed to do) from the market.

1914—Harrison Narcotics Act: Probably the most important legislation regarding opium. The act defined opium as a narcotic and was designed to control its sale.

1938—Food, Drug, and Cosmetics Act: This law required drug manufacturers to document and prove the safety of all their drugs and report their findings to the FDA.

1951—Durham-Humphrey Act: This law made the first distinction between prescription and nonprescription drugs. As a result, many medications could only be obtained through a physician's prescription.

1962—Kefauver-Harris Amendment: This law dealt with the effectiveness of new drugs. It required drug manufacturers to prove that their drugs were not only safe, but effective as well.

1970—Controlled Substances Act: This important piece of legislation outlines the control, evaluation, and penalties of all narcotic agents and other dangerous drugs.

U.S. LAW AND OPIUM

The control of opium by the U.S. government has continued to progress. Much of the legislation has been aimed at controlling the distribution and evaluating the safety and effectiveness of food and drugs in America. The story of U.S. opium law begins in 1905, when Congress officially banned opium, although the ban did little to stop physicians and patent medicine makers from selling opium in its many different forms. Just three years later, under increasing international drug legislation, the importation of opium for commercial use was banned. Opium could still be imported by the American pharmaceutical industry, which converted the raw opium into legitimate medicinal products. Despite these laws banning the importation and recreational use of opium, its use continued unabated across the country, until the passage of the Harrison Narcotics Act.

In 1914, there was an international outcry for the control of drug trafficking. A series of conventions on drug control (including the Shanghai Conference in 1909 and a conference at The Hague in 1911) led to the official agreement on the international control of opium in 1912. The U.S. Senate was finally ready to enact a domestic law to meet the newly formed international standards.

Although the 1914 Harrison Narcotics Act laid the groundwork for all future legislation regarding opium, it did not initially seem like a strict prohibition of the drug at all. With the official title—"An act to provide for the registration of, with collectors or internal revenue, and to impose a special tax upon all persons who produce, import, manufacture, compound, deal in, dispense, sell, distribute, or give away opium or coca leaves, their salts, derivatives, or preparations, and for other purposes"—the Harrison Narcotics Act was essentially about controlling opium providers. Only later was it reinterpreted to prohibit physicians and other people from distributing opium to addicts. After 1915, opium could no longer be easily obtained from a physician or pharmacist, nor in a laudanum product sold by a patent medicine maker.

One of the unforeseen offshoots of the Harrison Narcotics Act was the creation of an immense underground market. Realizing that the law had inadvertently enhanced the opium black market, a commission was appointed in 1918 to look into the matter. The commision found that the underground traffic in opium was equal to the legitimate trade, a national organization to distribute illicit opium had been established, and overall narcotics use had increased. Unfortunately, the legacy of drug law in the United States. is that it is never able to fully stop drug abuse. Many have accused the Harrison Narcotics Act of making the overall situation worse by forcing addicts into back alleys to buy opium and its constituents from peddlers. As a result of the drugs illegality, these vendors can now charge much more for the product than they could before. The Harrison Narcotics Act did make clear that more legislation would be required to establish any real control over opium.

MODERN DRUG CONTROL

Over the years, countless laws have been added or adjusted to deal with the changing drug culture in America, as the culture shifted from alcohol in the 1920s to psychedelic drugs in the 1960s. Throughout this time, opium derivatives, especially heroin, have remained a constant menace. The most important legislative action in recent history regarding drugs was the Controlled Substances Act (CSA) of 1971. Put into effect on May 1, 1971, the CSA was a sweeping law that replaced over 50 previous drug bills. The primary implication of the act was to create a single unified system for controlling both narcotics and psychedelics.

One important result of the CSA was the creation of a national list of narcotics and dangerous drugs that are federally controlled. The possession and trafficking of these drugs is strictly controlled by the federal government. The Controlled Substances List categorizes the most dangerous drugs into five "schedules" based on their danger to health, abuse potential, and medical uses. Generally, the potential for abuse and penalties decrease from Schedule I through Schedule V.

Another critical ramification of the CSA, and part of President Nixon's "war on drugs," was the creation of the Drug Enforcement Agency (DEA). At the time, one of the major

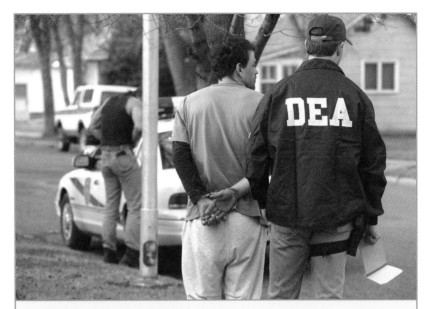

Figure 11.1 Drug Enforcement Administration (DEA) drug bust.
© Campbell William/CORBIS SYGMA

impediments to confronting the drug problem was the lack of coordination between various agencies, including the U.S. Customs Service and many local drug enforcement units, like the New York Drug Enforcement Task Force. The new DEA had broad authority to oversee the nation's drug policy and was given the authority to coordinate activities between all enforcement agencies.

OPIUM PENALTIES

Opium, as a rather complex drug with numerous forms used both medically and nonmedically, is scheduled by the DEA very specifically. Every aspect of the opium plant is considered a Schedule II controlled substance (Table 11.1). This means that it is illegal to possess or sell opium without a DEA license or prescription. More specifically, the DEA lists opium with the following wording:

1. Opium and opiate, and any salt, compound, derivative, or preparation of opium or opiate excluding apomorphine, thebaine-derived butorphanol, dextrorphan, nalbuphine, nalmefene, naxolone, and naltrexone, and their respective salts, but including the following:

THE FRENCH CONNECTION

From the late 1930s through the early 1970s, a vast underground network existed that was primarily responsible for supplying and increasing heroin abuse in the United States. During this period, the U.S. supply of licit opium used for medicines was coming from Turkey. However, the opium farmers in Turkey, along with selling their crops to pharmaceutical companies, often channeled excess product into the black market. The most common path that this excess opium took was by ship into one of the busiest international ports in the world—Marseilles, France. Once in port, the opium was taken to secret labs operated by Corsican gang leaders and converted into heroin. The heroin was then put back on ships bound for New York City. This process was called the "French Connection."

In the 1960s and 1970s, on average, drug enforcers seized about 200 pounds of heroin per year. This is a relatively unimpressive number when compared with the fact that this amount was shipped every other week. During this time, it is estimated that the French Connection was responsible for as much as 90 percent of the heroin consumed by addicts in the United States. The Connection flourished for many years, and it eventually took the combined forces of several nations' drug enforcement agencies to crack it. By 1972, through the efforts of narcotics agents from the United States, Italy, Canada, and France, the French Connection was all but destroyed.

      a. Raw Opium

      b. Opium Extracts

      c. Opium Fluid

      d. Powdered Opium

      e. Granulated Opium

      f. Tincture of Opium

2. Any salt, compound, derivative, or preparation thereof which is chemically equivalent or identical with any of the substances referred to in paragraph (b) (1) of this section, except that these substances shall not include the isoquinoline alkaloids of opium.

As evident by the preciseness of the DEA's wording concerning opium, every aspect of the drug is described. This was the result of distributors selling the drug in different forms (fluid, powdered, etc.) and claiming that it was legal. As a Schedule II drug, the legal ramifications of selling opium are severe. For example, a first offense equates to 10 years to life in prison or a $1 million to $4 million dollar fine (see Table 11.1). Penalties for possession of opium are less and vary depending on the amount in possession as well as individual state regulations. Nevertheless, getting caught in possession of opium is a serious matter.

THE FUTURE OF OPIUM

The story of opium is one that touches every part of the globe. It involves war, mass addiction, and international cooperation. Opium has created huge underground networks to supply the drug, which is mostly turned into heroin before being exported to the rest of the world. But the story of opium is also one of medical breakthroughs, as scientists have increasingly harnessed the drug's power to create useful drugs that have helped people cope with pain and numerous other medical ailments.

Table 11.1 Scheduling of Selected Opiates

Schedule	Potential for Abuse	Medical Use	Examples	Maximum Penalties for Trafficking*
I	High	None	Heroin, synthetic heroin, fentanyl (China white), morphine (pure forms)	*First offense:* 10 years to life in prison; $1 million to $4 million fine. *Second offense:* 20 years to life in prison; $2 million to $8 million fine. *2 or more prior offenses:* Life imprisonment
II	High	Yes	Codeine, morphine, meperidine (Demerol), opium poppy, opium tincture (Laudanum), granulated opium, powdered opium, raw opium, oxycodone (OxyContin, Percocet), thebaine	Same as Schedule I
III	Less than I and II	Yes	Codeine with papaverine or nescapine, opium combination product (Paragoric)	*First offense:* 5 years in prison; $250,000 fine. *Second offense:* 10 years in prison; $500,000 fine
IV	Low	Yes	Dextropropoxyphene dosage forms (Darvon, Propoxyphene, Darvocet)	NA
V	Lower than IV	Yes	Codeine preparations: 200 mg, 100 ml, or 100 gm (Robitussin)	NA

* These penalties represent the maximum possible trafficking punishments for most drugs in each respective schedule. Trafficking refers to the intent to distribute; penalties are generally less in possession cases. Many drugs, such as cocaine, heroin, and marijuana, have their own specific penalties. Penalties vary in relation to the quantity of drug involved.

Source: Drug Enforcement Agency (DEA), Available online. URL: http://www.usdoj.gov/dea/agency/penalties.htm. Accessed June 2, 2006.

Opium is a drug that has been used for thousands of years, and for all of these reasons, it will likely be used for thousands more. Using opium's various alkaloids, new drugs will be created and employed, just as new methods of consuming the drug may emerge. Governments are likely to increasingly cooperate to limit the production of the drug as it continues to handicap addicted populations. Opium, whether it is viewed as an angel or demon, medicine or dangerous narcotic, its story will continue as it always has, changing but not abating, into the distant future.

Glossary

acetylcholine—Neurotransmitter that relaxes the body.

alkaloids—Any of a host of organic compounds derived from plants; many are useful as medicines.

autocatalytic cycle—A cycle that fuels itself.

autonomic nervous system—The part of the nervous system responsible for unconscious actions, like heart rate. It is divided into two subparts: the sympathetic, responsible for activities that excite the body such as increasing respiration, and the parasympathetic, responsible for activities that relax the body such as lowering blood pressure.

central nervous system (CNS)—The brain and spinal cord; sensory nerve signals are sent to the CNS and it is responsible for many bodily activities, including movement and the release of chemical signals.

codeine—An alkaloid in opium used primarily as a cough suppressant.

detection period—The amount of time for which a drug test can detect the use of a drug (this differs depending on the type of sample—urine, blood, or other).

dihydrocodeine—A rather weak analgesic related to codeine, it is usually combined with other drugs and used as a headache suppressant.

dopamine—Neurotransmitter that causes euphoric feelings.

drug sensitivity—The amount of drug needed in a drug test sample to consider it a positive result.

epinephrine—Neurotransmitter that stimulates striated muscle, which is under conscious control.

fentanyl—A semi-synthetic opioid that is a much more powerful version of morphine. It is used during surgery as an anesthetic and is extremely dangerous when taken in a nonmedical context.

gas chromatography—A method for detecting the presence of illicit drugs in blood or urine. The sample is first inserted into the machine and vaporized (turned into a gas). As it vaporizes, different metabolites within the sample vaporize at different times, called retention times. The time differences are recorded and analyzed by the machine, which is pre-programmed to recognize the retention times of prohibited drugs.

heroin—A powerful, highly addictive narcotic made by boiling morphine; also known as diacetylmorphine.

hydrocodone—A widely prescribed, and abused, pharmaceutical designed as a pain-reliever.

hydromorphone—A pharmaceutical product used to combat severe pain.

immunoassays—A method for detecting the presence of illicit drugs in urine. Immunoassays involve the use of antibodies, proteins that can recognize and bind to a specific substance. To test for illegal opiate drugs, scientists find antibodies for the metabolite traces left by drugs in the urine. The urine and a solvent containing the antibodies are mixed together and scientists are then able to deduce if a drug is present by the reaction between the two substances.

laudanum—A mixture of opium and liquor once commonplace in English households.

mass spectrometry—A method for detecting the presence of illicit drugs in blood or urine. It uses an electron beam to separate the vaporized sample into its different ions according to their mass. The machine is able to separate all of the ions into groups and measure their concentrations. The metabolites for many enhancement drugs leave their own unique signature.

meperidine—Also known as pethidine, it is a synthetic opioid that is often used in place of morphine to treat pain.

methadone—A synthetic opioid that is commonly used today to treat heroin addicts.

morphine—Opium's most abundant alkaloid and active ingredient; used as a narcotic agent.

mules—The colloquial term for someone who smuggles illegal drugs on their person.

neurons—Nervous system cells with the specific job of transmitting signals to each other to coordinate a host of bodily functions.

neurotransmitters—Chemicals released by neurons to communicate with each other.

norepinephrine—Neurotransmitter that stimulates smooth muscles such as the heart and keeps blood pressure from lowering too much.

noscapine—A benzylisoquinoline alkaloid from opium that has only minimal medicinal and narcotic capabilities.

nostrums—Untested medications, produced by patent medicine makers, combining all kinds of natural products and drugs.

opioid receptors—A chemical lock-and-key mechanism located on cell surfaces that works because it allows only certain chemicals—in this case, opiates—to fit and thus communicate with the cell. There are three classifications of opioid receptors, mu, delta, and kappa.

opium—The narcotic drug obtained from the opium poppy; it is the oldest drug ever cultivated and actively pursued by the human species.

opium clippers—Ships developed in the mid-1800s specifically for the transport and sale of opium.

Glossary

opium den—An environ in which to smoke opium.

oxycodone—Derived from the alkaloid thebaine, it is a highly effective pain-reliever and prescribed to postsurgical patients, cancer patients, and others with severe pain.

papaverine—An alkaloid in opium with no narcotic properties used medicinally as a muscle relaxant.

Papaver somniferum—The opium poppy plant; it is one of only two species that produce morphine (the active ingredient in opium) and the only one actively cultivated to produce the drug.

parasympathetic system—The part of the autonomic nervous system responsible for activities that relax the body such as lowering blood pressure.

patent medicine makers—Unregulated small-time drug manufacturers prevalent in the nineteenth century.

poppy—The plant containing opium; a tall, thin plant of about 90–150 centimeters, its four sprouting leaves can be a variety of colors—white, pink, blue, crimson, or any combination of these—which surround the plant's inner pod.

propoxyphene—A synthetic opioid that is similar to methadone but much less potent.

serotonin—Neurotransmitter that inhibits bodily activities and acts as a counter to norepinephrine.

sympathetic system—The part of the autonomic nervous system responsible for activities that excite the body, such as increasing respiration.

synaptic cleft—The space between neurons.

thebaine—An alkaloid in opium that is actually a poison, causing convulsive effects when taken in high quantities.

Bibliography

Books

Berridge, Virginia, and Griffith Edwards. *Opium and the People*. New York: St Martin's Press, 1981.

Booth, Martin. *Opium: A History*. New York: St. Martin's Press, 1996.

Casy, Alan F., and Robert T. Partiff. *Opioid Analgesics: Chemistry and Receptors*. New York: Plenum Press, 1986.

Harding, Geoffrey. *Opiate Addiction, Morality and Medicine*. New York: St. Martin's Press, 1988.

Hodgson, Barbara. *Opium: Portrait of a Heavenly Demon*. San Francisco: Chronicle Books, 1999.

Moraes, Francis, and Debra Moraes. *Opium*. Oakland, Calif.: Ronin Publishing, 2003.

Rossi, S. (ed.). *Australian Medicines Handbook 2004*. Adelaide: Australian Medicines Handbook, 2004.

Articles, Websites, and Organizations

BLTC. "Endogenous Opioids." Available online at http://www.opioids.com/opiates.html. Accessed June 2, 2006.

Booth, Martin. "A Brief History of Opium." Available online at http://www.opioids.com/timeline. Accessed June 2, 2006.

Brecher, Edward. "The Consumers Union Report on Licit and Illicit Drugs, The Harrison Narcotic Act (1914)." Available online at http://www.druglibrary.org/schaffer/Library/studies/cu/cu8.html. Accessed June 2, 2006.

Drug Enforcement Agency. "Drug Scheduling." Available online at http://www.usdoj.gov/dea/pubs/scheduling.html. Accessed June 2, 2006.

Freevibe.com. "Misuse, Abuse, and Addiction." Available online at http://www.freevibe.com/Drug_Facts/prescription_misuse-abuse.asp. Accessed June 2, 2006.

Frontline. "The Opium Kings." *Public Broadcasting Service*. Available online at http://www.pbs.org/wgbh/pages/frontline/shows/heroin/etc/history.html. Accessed June 2, 2006.

Health World Online. "Detection of Opiates in Urine." Available online at http://www.healthy.net/clinic/lab/labtest/007.asp. Accessed June 2, 2006.

Humphreys, Keith. "Thomas De Quincey, *Confessions of an English Opium Eater*." *Addiction* 99:9 (2004): 1221–1222.

McCoy, Alfred W. "Opium History Up to 1858 A.D." Available online at http://www.opioids.com/opium/history/. Accessed June 2, 2006.

Bibliography

McCoy, Alfred W. "Opium History, 1979 to 1994." Available online at http://www.a1b2c3.com/drugs/opi012.htm. Accessed June 2, 2006.

Musto, David F. "The History of Legislative Control Over Opium, Cocaine, and Their Derivatives." *Schaffer Library of Drug Policy.* Available online at http://druglibrary.org/schaffer/history/ophs.htm. Accessed June 2, 2006.

National Drug Intelligence Center. "National Drug Threat Assessment 2005, Executive Summary: Heroin." Available online at http://www.usdoj.gov/ndic/pubs11/13745/heroin.htm. Accessed June 2, 2006.

Neer, Katherine. "How OxyContin Works." *How Stuff Works.* Available online at http://health.howstuffworks.com/oxycontin.htm/printable. Accessed June 2, 2006.

"Neuroscience for Kids—Heroin." Available online at http://faculty.washington.edu/chudler/hero.html. Accessed June 2, 2006.

NIDA (National Institute on Drug Abuse). "Mind Over Matter: The Brain's Response to Opiates." Available online at http://www.nida.nih.gov/MOM/OP/MOMOP1.html. Accessed June 2, 2006.

NIDA (National Institute on Drug Abuse). "NIDA InfoFacts: High School and Youth Trends." Available online at http://www.nida.nih.gov/Infofacts/HSYouthtrends.html. Accessed June 2, 2006.

NIDA (National Institute on Drug Abuse). "NIDA InfoFacts: Prescription Pain and Other Medication, Prescription Medications, Selected Prescription Drugs with Potential for Abuse." Available online at http://www.drugabuse.gov/infofacts/PainMed.html. Accessed June 2, 2006.

Partnership for a Drug-Free America. "Prescription Medicine Misuse and Abuse: A Growing Problem." Available online at http://www.drugfree.org/Portal/DrugIssue/Features/Prescription_Medicine_Misuse. Accessed June 2, 2006.

"Plant of Joy." Available online at http://www.opiates.net. Accessed June 2, 2006.

"Thomas De Quincey." Available online at http://www.kirjasto.sci.fi/quincey.htm. Accessed June 2, 2006.

U.S. Congress. Public Law No. 223, 63rd Congress, approved December 17, 1914.

United States Department of Justice. "History of the DEA: 1970–1975." Available online at http://www.dea.gov/pubs/history/1970-1975.html. Accessed June 2, 2006.

Vaults of Erowid. "Drug Testing Basics." Available online at http://www.erowid.org/psychoactives/testing/testing_info1.shtml. Accessed June 2, 2006.

Vaults of Erowid. "Opium—Legal Status." Available online at http://www.erowid.org/chemicals/opiates/opiates_law.shtml. Accessed June 2, 2006.

Waldman, Amy. "Afghan Route to Prosperity: Grow Poppies." *New York Times* (April 10, 2004)

Wikipedia.com. "Opioid Receptors." Available online at http://en.wikipedia.org/wiki/Opioid_receptor. Accessed June 2, 2006.

Further Reading

Books

Anonymous. *Go Ask Alice.* New York: Simon Pulse, 1998.

Beeching, Jack. *The Chinese Opium Wars.* New York: Harcourt, 1975.

Booth, Martin. *Opium: A History.* New York: St. Martin's Press, 1996.

De Quincey, Thomas. *Confessions of an English Opium Eater.* New York: Penguin, 2003.

Hodgson, Barbara. *Opium: Portrait of a Heavenly Demon.* San Francisco: Chronicle Books, 1999.

Tosches, Nick. *The Last Opium Den.* New York: Bloomsbury, 2002.

Web sites

Centers for Disease Control

http://www.cdc.gov

Drug Enforcement Administration

http://www.usdoj.gov/dea

Freevibe.com

http://www.freevibe.com

Frontline/ Public Broadcasting Service
"The Opium Kings"

http://www.pbs.org/wgbh/pages/frontline/shows/heroin/etc/history.html

How Stuff Works

http://howstuffworks.com

KidsHealth.org

http://www.kidshealth.org

Monitoring the Future Survey

http://www.monitoringthefuture.org

National Institute on Drug Abuse

http://www.nida.nih.gov

Office of National Drug Control Policy

http://www.whitehousedrugpolicy.gov

Opioids.com

http://www.opioids.com/index.html

Teendrugabuse.gov

http://www.teens.drugabuse.gov

Index

Index

Index

About the Author

Thomas M. Santella holds a Bachelor's degree in Secondary English Education and is pursuing a Master of History degree at Temple University. He is the Research Coordinator for Temple University's Center for Pharmaceutical Health Services Research, where he has collaborated with universities, governments, corporations, and aid organizations on a variety of health- and pharmaceutical-related projects. He has published work in a number of journals including *The Journal of Applied Research* and *The Journal of the American Pharmacists Association*, is a freelance writer and the author of *Body Enhancement Products*, and has traveled abroad to work on historical restoration projects. In addition to writing and research, he loves traveling, hiking, reading and music. He currently resides in Philadelphia, Pennsylvania.

About the Editor

David J. Triggle is a University Professor and a Distinguished Professor in the School of Pharmacy and Pharmaceutical Sciences at the State University of New York at Buffalo. He studied in the United Kingdom and earned his B.Sc. degree in Chemistry from the University of Southampton and a Ph.D. degree in Chemistry at the University of Hull. Following post-doctoral work at the University of Ottawa in Canada and the University of London in the United Kingdom, he assumed a position at the School of Pharmacy at Buffalo. He served as Chairman of the Department of Biochemical Pharmacology from 1971 to 1985 and as Dean of the School of Pharmacy from 1985 to 1995. From 1995 to 2001 he served as the Dean of the Graduate School, and as the University Provost from 2000 to 2001. He is the author of several books dealing with the chemical pharmacology of the autonomic nervous system and drug-receptor interactions, some 400 scientific publications, and has delivered over 1,000 lectures worldwide on his research.